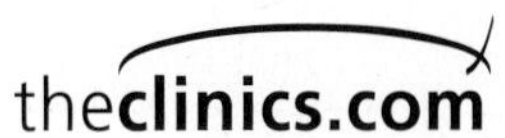

HEMATOLOGY/ ONCOLOGY CLINICS OF NORTH AMERICA

Sarcomas

GUEST EDITOR
Robert G. Maki, MD, PhD

June 2005 • Volume 19 • Number 3

SAUNDERS

An Imprint of Elsevier, Inc.
PHILADELPHIA LONDON TORONTO MONTREAL SYDNEY TOKYO

W.B. SAUNDERS COMPANY
A Division of Elsevier Inc.

Elsevier, Inc. • 1600 John F. Kennedy Boulevard • Suite 1800 • Philadelphia, Pennsylvania 19103-2899

http://www.theclinics.com

HEMATOLOGY/ONCOLOGY CLINICS OF NORTH AMERICA
June 2005
Editor: Kerry Holland

Volume 19, Number 3
ISSN 0889-8588
ISBN 1-4160-2774-2

Reprints. For copies of 100 or more, of articles in this publication, please contact the Commercial Reprints Department, Elsevier Inc., 360 Park Avenue South, New York, New York 10010-1710. Tel. (212) 633-3813 Fax: (212) 462-1935 email: reprints@elsevier.com

Hematology/Oncology Clinics of North America (ISSN 0889-8588) is published bi-monthly by W.B. Saunders Company. Corporate and editorial offices: Elsevier, Inc., 1600 John F. Kennedy Boulevard, Suite 1800, Philadelphia, PA 19103-2899. Accounting and circulation offices: 6277 Sea Harbor Drive, Orlando, FL 32887-4800. Periodicals postage paid at Orlando, FL 32862, and additional mailing offices. Subscription prices are $210.00 per year (US individuals), $315.00 per year (US institutions), $270.00 per year (foreign individuals), $380.00 per year (foreign institutions), $240.00 per year (Canadian individuals), and $380.00 per year (Canadian institutions). Foreign air speed delivery is included in all *Clinics* subscription prices. All prices are subject to change without notice. POSTMASTER: Send address changes to *Hematology/Oncology Clinics of North America,* W.B. Saunders Company, Periodicals Fulfillment, Orlando, FL 32887-4800. **Customer Service: 1-800-654-2452 (US). From outside the US, call 407-345-4000.** E-mail: hhspcs@harcourt.com

Hematology/Oncology Clinics of North America is covered in *Index Medicus, EMBASE/Excerpta Medica, and BIOSIS.*

Printed in the United States of America.

GUEST EDITOR

ROBERT G. MAKI, MD, PhD, Assistant Member, Department of Medicine; and Co-director, Adult Sarcoma Program, Memorial Sloan-Kettering Cancer Center, New York, New York

CONTRIBUTORS

KAREN H. ALBRITTON, MD, Chief, Adolescent and Young Adult Oncology Program; and Assistant Professor, Center for Sarcoma and Bone Oncology, Dana-Farber Cancer Institute and Harvard Medical School, Boston, Massachusetts

RICHARD CARVAJAL, MD, Fellow, Department of Medicine, Memorial Sloan-Kettering Cancer Center, New York, New York

EDWARD Y. CHENG, MD, Professor and Mairs Family Chair in Orthopaedic Oncology, Department of Orthopaedic Surgery, University of Minnesota; and Chief, Orthopaedic Surgery Service, Fairview-University Medical Center, Minneapolis, Minnesota

IAN JUDSON, MD, FRCP, Professor of Cancer Pharmacology, Cancer Research-UK Centre for Cancer Therapeutics, Institute of Cancer Research, Sutton, Surrey; and Consultant Medical Oncologist, Head of Sarcoma Unit, Royal Marsden NHS Foundation Trust, London, United Kingdom

ROBERT G. MAKI, MD, PhD, Assistant Member, Department of Medicine; and Co-director, Adult Sarcoma Program, Memorial Sloan-Kettering Cancer Center, New York, New York

IGOR MATUSHANSKY, MD, PhD, Memorial Sloan-Kettering Cancer Center, New York, New York

PAUL MEYERS, MD, Vice-Chairman, Department of Pediatrics, Memorial Sloan-Kettering Cancer Center, New York, New York

SHREYASKUMAR R. PATEL, MD, Professor, Department of Sarcoma Medical Oncology, The University of Texas, MD Anderson Cancer Center, Houston, Texas

MARCUS SCHLEMMER, MD, Medical Clinic and Polyclinic III, Clinic Grosshadern Munich, Ludwig-Maximilian-University Munich, Germany

SCOTT M. SCHUETZE, MD, PhD, Clinical Assistant Professor of Medicine, Division of Hematology/Oncology, University of Michigan Comprehensive Cancer Center, Ann Arbor, Michigan

MICHELLE SCURR, BMed, FRACP, Clinical Research Fellow, Cancer Research-UK Centre for Cancer Therapeutics, Institute of Cancer Research, Sutton, Surrey, United Kingdom

DEJKA M. STEINERT, MD, Medical Oncology Fellow, Division of Cancer Medicine, The University of Texas, MD Anderson Cancer Center, Houston, Texas

MARGARET VON MEHREN, MD, Member, Department of Medical Oncology, Fox Chase Cancer Center, Philadelphia, Pennsylvania

JAMES C. WATSON, MD, Associate Member, Department of Surgical Oncology, Fox Chase Cancer Center, Philadelphia, Pennsylvania

CONTENTS

FORTHCOMING ISSUES

August 2005

Primary Central Nervous System Lymphoma
Lisa DeAngelis, MD, and
Lauren Abrey, MD, *Guest Editors*

October 2005

Mesotheliomas
Hedy Kindler, MD, *Guest Editor*

December 2005

Sickle Cell Disease
Cage Johnson, MD, *Guest Editor*

RECENT ISSUES

April 2005

Multidisciplinary Approach to Lung Cancer
Gregory A. Masters, MD, FACP, FCCP, *Guest Editor*

February 2005

Antithrombotic Therapy: Current Practice and Future Trends
Rodger L. Bick, MD, PhD, FACP, *Guest Editor*

December 2004

Non-Malignant Disorders of the Blood in Infants and Children
George R. Buchanan, MD, *Guest Editor*

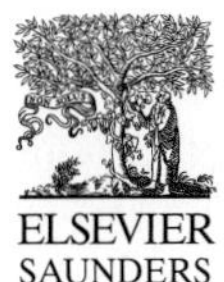

ELSEVIER
SAUNDERS

Hematol Oncol Clin N Am
19 (2005) xi–xii

HEMATOLOGY/
ONCOLOGY
CLINICS OF
NORTH AMERICA

Preface

Sarcomas

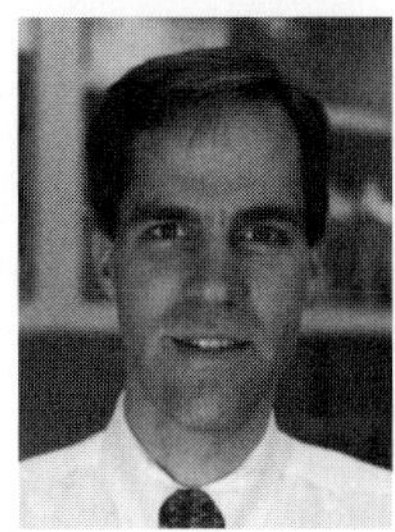

Robert G. Maki, MD, PhD
Guest Editor

It is with great pleasure that I introduce this volume of *Hematology-Oncology Clinics of North America* regarding the topic of sarcomas.

We are on the verge of dramatic changes in how cancer is diagnosed and treated. The labors of the molecular biologic revolution that have begun to break open the nature of the cancer cell of the last 50 years are beginning to bear fruit. There is no better evidence of this than the demonstration of the effectiveness of tyrosine kinase inhibitors such as imatinib and SU11248 in gastrointestinal stromal tumors. However, we are still faced with the finding that nearly half of people diagnosed with sarcomas of soft-tissue or bone will die of their disease. Pediatric studies have yielded one improvement after the next in the treatment of osteogenic sarcoma, Ewing sarcoma, and rhabdomyosarcoma, whereas much more modest gains have been seen for sarcomas typically observed in adults.

In pediatric, adolescent, and adult sarcomas, multimodality care is standard, and it is not unusual for surgeon, radiation oncologist, pathologist, and medical oncologist to collaborate closely to achieve the best possible outcome. You will find in this volume articles on aspects of the management and biology of sarcomas that represent the standard of care in 2005. Though it is a rapidly changing

This work was supported in part by NCI P01 grant CA47179.

0889-8588/05/$ – see front matter
doi:10.1016/j.hoc.2005.03.005

field, evidence-based analyses of clinical studies form the bedrock of the management of these diseases. The integration of new treatments with present-day management will be one of many challenges in the future for this group of tumors. It is my sincere hope the reader will find useful and timely information in the articles herein to help guide integration of old and new findings alike.

Robert G. Maki, MD, PhD
Memorial Sloan-Kettering Cancer Center
1275 York Avenue, Box 223
New York, NY 10021-6007, USA
E-mail address: makir@mskcc.org

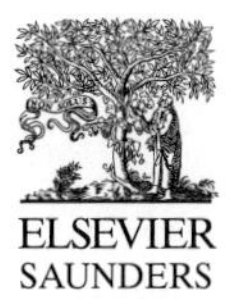
ELSEVIER
SAUNDERS

Hematol Oncol Clin N Am
19 (2005) 427–449

HEMATOLOGY/
ONCOLOGY
CLINICS OF
NORTH AMERICA

Mechanisms of Sarcomagenesis

Igor Matushansky, MD, PhD*, Robert G. Maki, MD, PhD

Memorial Sloan-Kettering Cancer Center, 1275 York Avenue, New York, NY 10021, USA

The word "sarcoma" dates to Galen (ca. 130–200) and the Greek term "σαρκωμα" describing a fleshy growth. Medically, sarcoma refers to those tumors that arise from mesenchymal cells—the same cells that lead to the formation of the connective tissues, such as bone, muscle, fat, cartilage, tendon, and ligaments [1]. Therefore, it is not surprising that for decades the classification system of sarcomas relied heavily on the tumors' resemblance to mature tissue. At the same time, the use of immunohistochemically defined antigens led to the proper diagnosis of difficult sarcoma lesions [2]. Immunohistochemical and genetic markers have been used to further define growth deregulation pathways in sarcomas [3]. More recently, the molecular classification of cancer has been prompted by the sequencing and annotation of the human genome and technical advancement in gene transcription profiling [4,5]. These scientific advancements provide insight into molecular pathways and mechanisms, which in turn clarify the biologic differences within soft-tissue sarcomas (STS) and pave the way for specific therapies for each STS subclass, if not for an individual patient's tumor.

There are approximately 10,000 new sarcoma cases each year in the United States, encompassing more than 50 different types of mesenchymal tumors (Boxes 1 and 2) [6]. Thus, the design of clinical trials aimed at studying a particular sarcoma subtype has been hindered by lack of sufficient patient accrual per histopathologic diagnosis. Fortunately, clinical correlative data indicate that molecular analysis is more important than site of origin in terms of treatment options and prognosis [7–10], enforcing the need for further molecular studies.

This work was supported in part by the Sarcoma Program Project Grant CA 47179, the Harris Family Foundation, and the Abraham and Phyllis Katz Foundation.

* Corresponding author.

E-mail address: matushai@mskcc.org (I. Matushansky).

doi:10.1016/j.hoc.2005.03.006

hemonc.theclinics.com

Box 1. Histologic classification of malignant sarcomas (soft tissue sarcomas)

Fibrous tumors
- Adult fibrosarcoma
- Inflammatory fibrosarcoma

Fibrohistiocytic tumors
- Malignant fibrous histiocytoma (MFH, now termed undifferentiated high-grade pleomorphic sarcoma)
  - Storiform-pleomorphic
  - Myxoid (myxofibrosarcoma)
  - Giant cell (malignant giant cell tumor of soft parts)
  - Inflammatory

Lipomatous tumors
- Well-differentiated liposarcoma
  - Lipoma-like liposarcoma
  - Sclerosing liposarcoma
  - Inflammatory liposarcoma
- Dedifferentiated liposarcoma
- Myxoid/round cell liposarcoma
- Pleomorphic liposarcoma

Smooth muscle tumors
- Leiomyosarcoma
- Epithelioid leiomyosarcoma

Skeletal muscle tumors
- Rhabdomyosarcoma
  - Embryonal rhabdomyosarcoma
  - Botryoid rhabdomyosarcoma
  - Spindle cell rhabdomyosarcoma
  - Alveolar rhabdomyosarcoma
  - Pleomorphic rhabdomyosarcoma
  - Rhabdomyosarcoma with ganglionic differentiation (ectomesenchymoma)

Tumors of blood and lymph vessels
- Epithelioid hemangioendothelioma
- Angiosarcoma and lymphangiosarcoma
- Kaposi sarcoma

Perivascular tumors
- Malignant glomus tumor (glomangiosarcoma)
- Malignant hemangiopericytoma/solitary fibrous tumor

Giant cell tumors
- Malignant giant cell tumor of tendon sheath

Neural tumors
- Malignant peripheral nerve sheath tumor (MPNST, neurofibrosarcoma)
  - Malignant Triton tumor (MPNST with rhabdomyosarcoma)
  - Glandular MPNST
  - Epithelioid MPNST

Extraskeletal cartilaginous and osseous tumors
- Extraskeletal chondrosarcoma
  - Extraskeletal myxoid chondrosarcoma
  - Mesenchymal chondrosarcoma
- Extraskeletal osteosarcoma

Pluripotential mesenchymal tumors
- Malignant mesenchymoma

Miscellaneous tumors
- Alveolar soft part sarcoma
- Epithelioid sarcoma
- Malignant extrarenal rhabdoid tumor
- Desmoplastic small round cell tumor (DSRCT)
- Ewing sarcoma/Primitive neuroectodermal tumor
- Extraskeletal Ewing sarcoma
- Clear cell sarcoma (melanoma of soft parts)
- Gastrointestinal stromal tumors
- Synovial sarcoma
  - Biphasic synovial sarcoma
  - Monophasic synovial sarcoma

Considered from a molecular point of view, sarcomas can be divided into two major classes. The first involves sarcomas with specific aberrancies in known cell cycle regulatory pathways (Rb, p53, and so forth, or their upstream/downstream targets). The second involves sarcomas with either simple or complex karyotypes and resulting chromosomal translocations and aneuploidy, respectively. This review discusses in general some of the aberrant molecular mechanisms shared in sarcomas as well as several subtypes of sarcomas in which the most advances have been made. Finally, the ways in which these advances in basic science translate into and redefine clinical practice are highlighted.

Sarcomas and cell cycle regulatory proteins

General concepts

Disruption in genes that control cell cycle regulation affects at least three different types of genes in sarcomas. The first type involves genes that

Box 2. Histologic classification of malignant sarcomas (sarcomas of bone and cartilage)

- *Intramedullary osteosarcoma*
  - Telangiectatic
  - Well-differentiated (low-grade intraosseous)
  - Conventional
    - Osteoblastic
    - Chondroblastic
    - Fibroblastic
    - Malignant fibrous histiocytoma (MFH)-like
    - Osteoblastoma-like
    - Giant cell-rich
    - Small cell
    - Epithelioid
- *Surface osteogenic sarcoma*
  - Parosteal (juxtacortical)
  - Periosteal
  - High-grade surface (de novo and dedifferentiated)
- *Intracortical osteogenic sarcoma*
- *Chondrosarcoma*
  - Intramedullary
  - Conventional type
  - Dedifferentiated
  - Clear-cell
  - Mesenchymal
  - Juxtacortical
- *Malignant fibrous histiocytoma (MFH) of bone*
- *Fibrosarcoma of bone*
- *Giant cell tumor of bone*
  - Conventional type
  - Multifocal conventional giant cell tumor
  - Conventional giant cell tumor with lung metastases
  - Malignant giant cell tumor
    - Secondary
    - Primary
- *Vascular sarcomas of bone*
  - Epithelioid hemangioendothelioma
  - Angiosarcoma
- *Cystic lesions*
  - Aneurysmal bone cyst
- *Smooth muscle sarcomas affecting bone*
  - Leiomyosarcoma of bone

Synovial tumors
- Synovial chondromatosis
- Synovial chondrosarcoma
- Pigmented villonodular synovitis

Bone sarcomas of uncertain origin
- Ewing sarcoma/Primitive neuroectodermal tumor (PNET)
- Malignant mesenchymoma
- Adamantinoma
  - Classic
  - Differentiated (osteofibrous dysplasia-like)
- Chordoma
  - Conventional
  - Chondroid
  - Dedifferentiated

mediate signals from the cell surface to the cell nucleus. A constitutively active signal transduction cascade, which has been observed in several sarcoma subtypes, leads to continuous proliferation of cells, presumably predisposing these cells to further genetic mutations that result in mesenchymal cell transformation at an early phase of differentiation and sarcoma formation. The second type involves mutations in genes that control progression through the cell cycle and are the effector arms of the signal transduction cascade. This group of genes is most notably represented by the retinoblastoma tumor suppressor protein (pRb). The third type involves mutations in genes responsible for maintaining DNA integrity on replication. This group of genes is most notably represented by the p53 tumor suppressor protein. Please refer to Fig. 1 for a schematic representation.

Signal transduction

Disruption in signal transduction can be divided into two types, those involving constitutive activation of signal transduction cascades via known mechanisms and those involving unknown mechanisms.

A classic example of a sarcoma with constitutive activation of a signal transduction cascades via a known mechanism is the fusion of the transcription factor ETV6 with growth factor receptor tyrosine kinase NTRK3 [11] in congenital fibrosarcomas leading to constitutive activation of the NTRK3-receptor signaling pathway. This specific fusion occurs due to a translocation between chromosomes 12 and 15 [t(p2;15)(p13;q25)]. As stated previously, this constitutive activation leads to a hyperproliferative state, which on fulfillment of Knudson's hypothesis (ie, a second genetic event [12]) leads to sarcomagenesis.

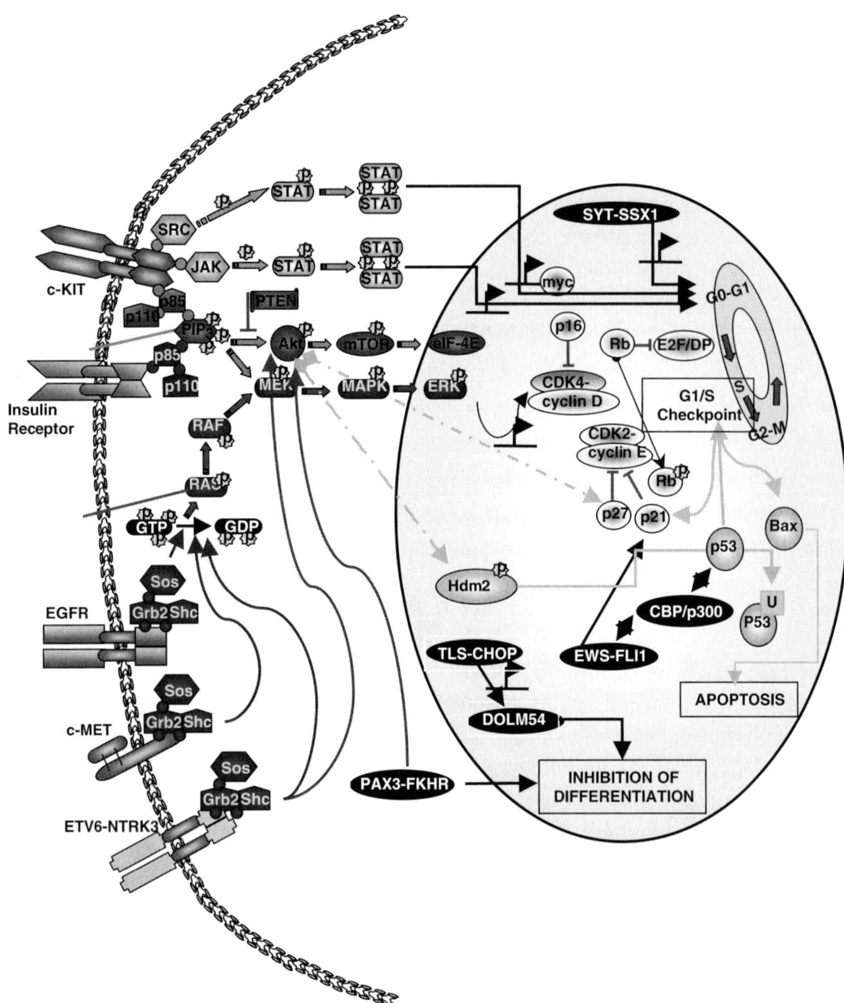

Fig. 1. Schematic representation of major pathways known to be involved in sarcomagenesis. (See text for full details.)

On the other hand, activation of the c-Met receptor pathway seen in synovial sarcomas [13] occurs via unclear mechanisms. Synovial sarcoma is an aggressive spindle cell sarcoma occurring predominantly in young adults. At the genetic level, synovial sarcoma is characterized in over 95% of cases by a specific chromosomal translocation, t(X;18)(p11.2;q11.2), which juxtaposes the SYT gene on chromosome 18 to either the SSX1 (60%) or the SSX2 gene (40%) on chromosome X. Although the exact activation mechanism is unclear, the chimeric SYT-SSX product is thought to function as a transcriptional protein that deregulates gene expression, thereby providing a putative growth stimulus [14]. Additionally, c-MET, a proto-oncogene [15], has been shown to be activated in synovial sarcomas [13]. While the relationship between SYT-SSX and activation of the c-Met receptor pathway activation is unclear, their cooperation, as based on clinicopathologic correlation [13], suggests that c-MET signaling may contribute to tumorigenesis and progression in synovial sarcoma.

Although the exact mechanisms by which dysregulation of cellular signaling leads to specific dysregulation at the transcriptional level that results in cellular transformation is unknown, a common point of convergence in many signal transduction pathways affected in sarcomas appears to be the PI3K-AKT pathway [16]. AKT is activated by multiple cell surface receptors and in turn can activate multiple downstream signal transduction cascades, thus connecting the stimulus of cell surface receptors to the activation and inhibition of transcriptional targets, resulting in cellular survival, growth, and proliferation through distinct mechanisms. As discussed later, elucidation of these pathways and the means by which to inhibit them is rapidly becoming more than just a molecular biology exercise, as elements of each pathway immediately represent targets for therapeutic interventions.

Retinoblastoma tumor suppressor protein pathway

Multiple lines of evidence implicate retinoblastoma tumor suppressor protein (pRb) in sarcomagenesis: (1) the majority of sarcomas have alterations in the Rb pathway; (2) patients with hereditary retinoblastoma are at an increased risk of developing sarcomas [17]; (3) patients with single gene Rb defects have an increased risk of developing sarcomas upon radiation exposure [18].

The product encoded by the RB gene (pRb) has been identified as a critical cell cycle regulator [19]. pRb is the key regulator of the G1/S transition, acting as a transcriptional repressor when bound to proteins from the E2F family. pRb phosphorylation is tightly controlled by cyclin D1/Cdk4 and secondarily by the cyclin-dependent kinase inhibitors. In transformed cells, animal models, and human cancers, alterations, manifested by either point mutations (activating or inhibitory) or chromosomal changes (amplification or deletion), have been shown to contribute to tumorigenesis [20]. Each of these events contributes to hyperphosphorylation of pRB and disruption of the G1/S transition in a manner analogous to Rb mutation. Not unexpectedly, cyclin D1 overexpression is a frequent event in adult soft tissue sarcomas and is associated with high grade tumors and poor survival [21]. Amplification and overexpression of CDK4, mapping to 12q13-14, a region frequently amplified in human tumors, is a common event in osteosarcoma and well-differentiated and dedifferentiated liposarcoma and associated with metastatic potential [22]. Furthermore, the cyclin-dependent kinase inhibitor p16 is often inactivated in STS, a phenomenon associated with aggressive biologic behavior and poor outcome [7].

p53 tumor suppressor protein pathway

The transcription factor p53 has been called the guardian of the genome [23] and has been observed to be mutated in 60% of all sarcomas [24]. In essence it serves two functions: (1) p53 senses DNA damage and mediates prolongation of G1-arrest to provide sufficient time to repair DNA damage, and (2) p53 also mediates apoptosis when DNA damage is deemed unrepairable [25]. Transcriptional targets of p53 include intrinsic apoptotic regulators such as Bax, Noxa, Puma and Bid; as well as extrinsic regulators, such as Fas [26]. More recently, it has been shown that p53 is able to induce apoptosis in a transcription-independent manner. Such process is initiated in the cytosol, might be controlled by Hdm2 levels, and requires p53 localization in the mitochondria [27]. HDM2 (human MDM2) amplification is frequently observed in well-differentiated and dedifferentiated liposarcomas and malignant fibrous histiocytomas [28]. After DNA damage, p53 is mobilized to the mitochondria and binds to Bcl-X_L, thus liberating pro-apoptotic proteins such as Bid. This mitochondrial localization of p53 also triggers Bax oligomerization, which in turn causes cytochrome c release leading to apoptosis. Bcl-2, an antagonist of Bax pro-apoptotic function, is overexpressed and associated with the clinical aggressiveness of synovial sarcomas [29]. In a series of retrospective analyses, p53 nuclear accumulation has been shown to be a prognostic determinant in adult sarcomas [30]. Specifically, desmoid tumors and fibrosarcomas are part of a wide spectrum of disordered fibroblastic growth that displays striking clinical and phenotypic differences. There was a trend for an increasing abnormal expression of p53 paralleling tumor aggressiveness from desmoid tumors to low grade fibrosarcoma to high grade fibrosarcoma [31]. Finally, from an historical perspective, the index case for the original family with Li-Fraumeni syndrome (caused by p53 mutations) had rhabdomyosarcoma [32].

The Rb-p53-Akt axis

One can envision the following model of sarcomagenesis: independence of growth factor control is attained by dysregulation in the signal transduction cascade by means differing and specific to each sarcoma subtype. Akt, central to the signal transduction cascade, mediates the constitutively active signal leading to hyperproliferation. Secondary genetic alterations than occur as a consequence of the hyperproliferative state (eg, p53 and Rb pathway mutations) that result in a further selective advantage to these cells. With the addition of further genetic changes, inhibition of differentiation ensues. The end product of this process is a transformed cell. One could also envision how this process could begin with differentiation arrest (either as a response to specific growth factor autonomy needed for differentiation or the direct result of a transcriptionally active fusion gene product) and then other secondary events occur that provide a selective advantage to allow the differentiation-arrested cell to proliferate in its immature state.

Sarcomas and karyotype abnormalities

General concepts

Cytogenetically sarcomas fall into two broad groups [8]: (1) sarcomas with specific genetic alterations and usually simple karyotypes, including reciprocal translocations that result in fusion genes; and (2) sarcomas with nonspecific genetic alterations and complex unbalanced karyotypes, evidenced by numerous chromosomal losses and gains.

Table 1
A selection of chromosomal changes observed in soft-tissue sarcoma

Tumor histology	Chromosomal alteration	Involved gene(s)	Frequency (%)
Ewing sarcoma family[a]	t(11;22)(q24;q12)	EWS-FLI1	85
	t(21;22)(q22;q12)	EWS-ERG	5–10
	t(7;22)(p22;q12)	EVT1-EWS	Rare
	t(17;22)(q12;q12)	EIAF-EWS	Rare
	t(1;16)(q11-25;q11-24)	Unknown	~10
	Trisomy 8	Not applicable	~50
	Trisomy 12	Not applicable	~30
Myxoid/round cell liposarcoma	t(12;16)(q13;p11)	TLS (FUS)-CHOP	>75
	t(12;22)(q13;q12)	EWS-CHOP	Uncommon
Atypical lipomatous tumor/well differentiated liposarcoma	12q rings and giant markers	HMGIC, CDK4, and MDM2 amplification	60
Alveolar rhabdomyosarcoma	t(2;13)(q35;q14)	PAX3-FKHR	~70
	t(1;13)(p36;q14)	PAX7-FKHR	~15
Clear cell sarcoma (melanoma of soft parts)	t(12;22)(q13;q12)	EWS-ATF1	>75
Desmoplastic small round cell tumor (DSRCT)	t(11;22)(p13;q12)	EWS-WT1	>90
Synovial sarcoma	t(X;18)(p11;q11)	SYT-SSX1, SYT-SSX2	>90
Extraskeletal myxoid chondrosarcoma	t(9;22)(q22;q12)	EWS-CHN (TEC)	>75
Dermatofibrosarcoma protuberans (DFSP)	t(17;22)(q22;q13), ring chromosomes	COL1A1-PDGFB	>50; ring chromosomes >75
Congenital fibrosarcoma	t(12;15)(p13;q25)	ETV6 (TEL)-NTRK3 (TRKC)	Unknown
Malignant rhabdoid tumor	del 22(q11.2)	hSNF5/INI1	~50[b]

[a] Ewing family of tumors includes Ewing sarcoma, PNET (peripheral neuroectodermal tumor), and Askin tumor.

[b] Mutations seen in other cases, giving >80% with disruption of the hSNF5 gene.

Sarcomas with simple karyotypes

Sarcomas with simple karyotypes are characterized by specific recurrent chromosomal translocations that produce specific gene fusion products pathognomonic for a specific sarcoma subtype (Table 1). These fusion products encode for either transcription factors (eg, Ewing sarcoma [33]) or growth factors (eg, dermatofibrosarcoma protuberans [34]). Generally, these are each thought to deregulate the expression of specific repertoires of downstream target genes, possibly providing multiple oncogenic hits analogous to the multistep process of epithelial carcinogenesis. So far, secondary mutations have been identified in many of these sarcomas [35] but none have been shown to be necessary for tumorigenesis. However, this generality fails to explain the specificity of the translocation to the corresponding sarcoma. To date three theories have been brought forward regarding the association between specific translocations and corresponding sarcomas. The first theory states that the translocation product determines the tumor type regardless of the cell of origin. The second theory states that cell type and its stage of differentiation leads to tumorigenesis in the presence of an oncogene, regardless of the specific fusion product. Finally the third theory states that even though the translocation might be a rare event in any one cell type, only cells at specific points in the mesenchymal differentiation program are both susceptible to and permissive of the effects of a given fusion gene. This is currently an active area of investigation.

Sarcomas with complex karyotypes

Sarcomas with complex karyotypes are characterized by extensive cytogenetic abnormalities (eg, malignant fibrous histiocytoma, Box 3). These include chromosomal deletions, amplifications, gains and losses of whole chromosomes, and aneuploidy [36]. Although there is an association between cumulative chromosomal abnormalities and high-grade tumors [8], there does not seem to be a consistency to the genetic damage within a tumor subtype and the finding of multiple and complex genetic abnormalities in these sarcoma subtypes makes identifying the contribution of any one abnormality difficult. Furthermore, although chromosomal instability, as measured by aneuploidy, is observed in nearly all solid tumors [36], its contributions to tumorigenesis as well as the molecular defects leading to it in cancer cells are less clear [37].

In fact, the issue of whether aneuploidy itself is a cause or a consequence of the malignant phenotype is also still unclear in tumors [38]. The latter, also known as the "aneuploid theory of cancer origin" first proposed by Theodor Boveri almost a century ago [39], continues to be highly debated in the literature [40,41]. Thus, it is possible that at least some of the complex chromosomal gains and losses may simply reflect the marked genomic instability innate to certain sarcomas and may not directly contribute to tumorigenesis. Recently there has been some clarification regarding this fundamental issue. Human tumors have two mechanisms by which telomere length can be maintained: telomerase

Box 3. Sarcomas with complex karyotypes

- Fibrosarcoma
- Leiomyosarcoma
- High-grade undifferentiated pleomorphic sarcoma (malignant fibrous histiocytoma, MFH)
- Osteosarcoma
- Chondrosarcoma
- Liposarcoma
  - Well differentiated/dedifferentiated (ring, giant, and marker chromosomes)
  - Pleomorphic liposarcoma
- Rhabdomyosarcoma
  - Embryonal
  - Pleomorphic
- Malignant peripheral nerve sheath tumor (MPNST, malignant schwannoma, neurofibrosarcoma)
- Angiosarcoma

activation and alternative lengthening of telomeres (ALT). A study of these mechanisms in sarcomas indicated that sarcomas with simple karyotypes used telomerase activation, whereas sarcomas with complex karyotypes used ALT [42]. This observed dichotomy suggests that telomere dysfunction might serve two different functions in sarcomagenesis. In the complex karyotype sarcomas, aneuploidy might promote tumor progression leading to accumulation of genetic changes that are representative of the full malignant phenotype, highly reminiscent of the model of tumorigenesis in telomerase-null mice [43]. In the simple karyotype sarcomas, accumulation of chromosomal abnormalities may be disadvantageous since the transforming event, represented by the fusion gene, has already occurred [44]. Further genetic changes could be as likely disrupt the oncogenic mechanism as they are to promote it; however, some of these genetic events are the force providing some of the tumor cells with a selective advantage for their survival.

Molecular mechanisms of specific sarcoma subtypes

Liposarcoma

Liposarcoma is the most common STS and accounts for approximately 20% of all mesenchymal malignancies. Previous histologic classification has divided liposarcomas into five histologic subtypes: well differentiated, dedifferentiated, myxoid, round cell, and pleomorphic. All five exhibit unique biologic behaviors

[45]. Due to recent advances in genetic profiling and chromosomal analysis, liposarcomas can be reclassified into three types:

Liposarcomas characterized by ring or long marker chromosomes derived from the long arm of chromosome 12, consisting predominantly of the dedifferentiated type

Amplification of sequences from the 12q14-15 chromosome region results in amplification of HDM2 (human MDM2) and CDK4 [46,47], both of which have been implicated in the tumorigenesis of other malignancies. HDM2 functions to negatively regulate p53 expression by targeting p53 for degradation; thus overexpression of HDM2 can lead to a p53 null-like state and predisposition to tumor formation [48]. Overexpression of CDK4 maintains Rb in the hyper-phosphorylated state, preventing Rb from inhibiting E2F–mediated cell cycle progression. This latter state is analogous to cells with Rb mutations [20]. These genes might provide the transformation potential, whereas other genes amplified on chromosome 12 may determine the cell type and stage of differentiation. Putative genes in this regard include HMGA2 (a gene involved in adipocyte differentiation [49] and GLI (a putative oncogene involved in the sonic hedgehog signaling pathway and embryonic tissue specificity [50].

Liposarcomas characterized by a reciprocal translocation t(12;16)(q13;p11), consisting of myxoid and round cell (poorly differentiated myxoid) types

Myxoid and round cell liposarcoma accounts for about 30% to 35% of all liposarcomas and share significant clinical and morphologic features. Tumors displaying both types concurrently are often seen [51] leading to the concept that round cell liposarcoma is the high grade component of myxoid liposarcoma [45]. This notion is strongly supported by the fact that myxoid and round cell liposarcoma share the same characteristic chromosomal change, a reciprocal translocation t(12;16)(q13;p11) that fuses full length CHOP gene with the N-terminus of the TLS gene. CHOP is a transcription factor involved in the regulation of the cell cycle and apoptosis in response to cellular stress [52]. TLS is an RNA/DNA-binding protein [53]. Thus it is hypothesized that TLS changes the specificity of CHOP target genes leading to tumorigenesis [54]. This notion is supported by the finding of DOL54 ("downstream of the gene for the liposarcoma-associated fusion oncoprotein 54"), a gene involved in adipocytic differentiation and specifically activated by TLS/CHOP fusion proteins but not by CHOP [55]. Activation of DOL54 may provide cell type and stage specificity, which in the presence of other genetic events yet to be identified may lead to transformation.

Liposarcomas characterized by complex karyotypes, predominantly represented by pleomorphic liposarcomas and well-differentiated liposarcomas

Liposarcomas exhibit stable supernumerary giant and ring chromosomes. Structurally abnormal chromosomes are usually unstable because they lack functional centromeres (acentric chromosomes) as measured by the absence of alpha-satellite (or alphoid) sequences which appear adjacent to the centromere of all normal human chromosomes [56]. Recently, stable chromosomes lacking alpha-satellite sequences, called analphoid chromosomes, have been identified, and well-differentiated liposarcoma is the first example of a tumor class for which the presence of stable analphoid chromosomes is a characteristic abnormality [57]. In the absence of a functional centromere, the mechanism by which these cells are able to proliferate remains unclear. One explanation is that centromere function can be acquired by other means such as changes in acetylation status of chromatin, of shift in the replication timing at unusual sites, alterations in the acetylation pattern of centromeric chromatin, and targeting of specific protein-protein interactions mediated by CENPA or CENPC (reviewed in [58]). These adaptive mechanisms would then lead to "neo-centromere" activation and thus provide a selective advantage to neoplastic cells for replication of genetically aberrant material. Specific targeting of neo-centromere formation represents a novel target for therapeutics.

Alveolar rhabdomyosarcoma

Alveolar rhabdomyosarcoma (ARMS) is a subtype of rhabdomyosarcoma (RMS), a family of pediatric soft tissue tumors that are related to the skeletal muscle lineage [59]. RMS is exceedingly infrequent in adult. The most prevalent finding in ARMS is a translocation, t(2;13)(q35-37;q14), which results in a chimeric transcript composed of 5′ PAX3 sequences fused to 3′ FKHR sequences [60]. PAX3 is a member of the paired-box family of transcription factors, which direct various developmental processes, and has distinct functions in the developing neural crest and muscle [61]. The fusion partner, FKHR (now termed FOXO1A), is a ubiquitously expressed member of the forkhead family of transcription factors. Its normal function is regulated through phosphorylation by AKT, and it is thought to regulate genes that are related to apoptosis [62]. In the PAX3–FKHR fusion, the DNA-binding domain of FKHR is lost, and therefore any DNA-binding specificity of the fusion gene is directed by the PAX3 sequences. The fusion product has been shown to both promote early myogenic differentiation but inhibit terminal differentiation in cell culture models, suggesting that PAX3–FKHR may arrest the differentiating cell at a specific point in the differentiation pathway at which it is susceptible to transformation mediated by further genetic events [63]. The simultaneous interaction of PAX3–FKHR with the AKT pathway might provide the basis for further genetic changes as discussed above. Alternatively, activation of the IGF signaling pathway is well documented in ARMS and evidence of cooperativity between PAX3–FKHR and IGF2 in models of rhabdomyosarcoma have been observed [64].

Ewing sarcoma

Ewing sarcoma is the second most common malignant bone tumor occurring in children and young adults, and accounts for 10% to 15% of all primary bone tumors [65]. The t(11;22)(q24;q12) chromosome rearrangement has become pathognomonic for this tumor [66], although there are variants of this translocation seen in a subset of patients. The translocation leads to aberrant fusion of the RNA-binding protein EWS on chromosome 22 to the juxtaposed to the DNA-binding ETS transcriptional factor Fli-1 on chromosome 11 [67]. Several lines of evidence indicate that EWS/FLI-1 related fusion proteins are necessary and sufficient to induce transformation both in vivo and in vitro. Transduction of EWS/FLI-1 into NIH 3T3 cells to display contact-independent growth that is characteristic of cellular transformation [68]. Thus the EWS/Fli-1 fusion protein functions in part as a chimeric transcription factor contributing to malignant transformation via transactivation of FLI-1 target genes. However, while multiple potential target genes have been identified, little evidence exists to date demonstrating that these genes are consistently deregulated in Ewing sarcoma. The most obvious target of EWS-Fli-1 is the p21 cyclin-dependent kinase inhibitor, resulting in p21 gene suppression and a phosphorylated Rb [69]. p21 has been implicated in tumorigenesis in several other cancer models [20]. However, p21 does not appear to be suppressed in all the Ewing sarcoma samples [70], indicating that alternative mechanisms must exist. One such mechanism may be interaction of the EWS-Fli-1 protein with CBP [71]. CBP/p300 functions as a coactivator for numerous transcriptional factors and interacts with general transcriptional factors such as TBP and TFIID acting as a link to transcriptional machinery [72]. This interaction might lead to sequestration of CBP from p53, leading to deregulation of apoptotic control during cellular replication. Along this theme, it has been shown that: (1) exogenous expression of EWS/Fli-1 protein in primary human fibroblasts result in induction of p53 and cell cycle arrest; and (2) abrogation of the p53 pathway prevents growth suppression [73]. Taken together these results suggest that p53 loss of function is a necessary event for Ews/Fli-1 to cause tumorigenesis and that EWS-Fli-1 might act as anti-apoptotic agents through targeting the CBP/p300 pathways. Inhibition of known downstream mediators of apoptosis in this setting might lead to a better understanding of this sarcoma subtype.

Gastrointestinal stromal tumors

Gastrointestinal stromal tumors (GISTs) are mesenchymal neoplasms characterized by the expression of the receptor tyrosine kinase KIT (CD117) [8]. Recent studies have established that activating mutations of KIT are present in up to 92% of GISTs and likely lead to constitutive activation of the kinase and transformation [74,75]. GISTs appear to originate from interstitial cells of Cajal (ICCs), pacemaker cells for the autonomous contraction of the gastrointestinal tract [76]. Specifically, both GISTs and ICCs simultaneously express KIT and CD34, and multiple GISTs appear to develop from diffuse ICC hyperplasia in the background of a germ line mutation in the c-kit gene. Because somatic gain-of-function mutations of the c-kit gene are observed in solitary GISTs and familial and multiple GISTs, the gain-of-function mutations of the c-kit gene are considered to be a cause of the formation of GISTs [77].

Although the discovery of stem cell factor (SCF) and its receptor (Kit) occurred almost 25 years ago [78], its mode of action and mechanism by which its constitutive activation leads to transformation continues to be elucidated. c-Kit can act synergistically with other growth factor receptors to promote survival, proliferation, and differentiation of multiple cellular lineages [79]. Signaling through the c-kit receptor can be separated into three pathways that result in transcriptional gene control. These pathways are: (1) Raf-1/MAP kinase; (2) induction of c-myc through activation of src or other src family members; and (3) activation of the Janus family of protein tyrosine kinases. Further molecular characterization reveals that specific mutations in c-kit receptor result in differential regulation of these pathways, which, in the background of the appropriate milieu (ie, ICC in the case of GIST), leads to transformation.

Sarcoma and targeted therapy

Rapid advances in understanding the molecular mechanisms in sarcomagenesis have led to the development of new biologic agents based on the specific biology of specific sarcomas. These agents, some already in current practice, are truly exemplary models of targeted therapy and the standard by which future targeted therapy will be measured. This section briefly discusses such developments from an overall point of view as well as with some specific examples.

Conceptual approaches

Targeting signal transduction cascades

The mammalian target of rapamycin (mTOR) is a member of the phosphoinositide 3-kinase–related kinase family and a central modulator of cellular signaling pathways connecting extracellular stimulus via insulin, nutrients, and growth factors to the translational machinery of the cell leading to ribosomal biosynthesis and translation of key mRNAs of proteins as required for G1 to S phase progression [80,81]. Insulin signaling through the insulin-like growth factor (IGFR)-mTOR pathway has been shown to be important in the differentiation of progenitor cells along multiple mesenchymal lineages [82,83]. Additionally, IGFR has been found to be overexpressed in several sarcoma subtypes including Ewing sarcoma [84] and synovial sarcoma [85]. Finally, activation of the IGF signaling pathway has been well documented in ARMS and evidence of cooperativity between PAX3–FKHR and IGF2 in models of rhabdomyosarcoma has been observed [64]. Taken together, there is good rationale for the development of mTOR pathway inhibitors for the treatment of sarcomas. This rationale is further supported by the observation that CCI-779, an mTOR inhibitor, acts additively with an IGF binding protein in a rhabdomyosarcoma cell culture and xenograft mouse model system [86]. Although, clinical trials are in progress and have not specifically addressed the efficacy of CCI-779 in sarcoma, preclinical data are encouraging because they provide additional evidence that might indicate that tumors, such as sarcomas, which are more developmentally dependent on the insulin-IGFR-mTOR pathway, might show greater clinical responses. However, the complexity of the cascades flowing into and out of Akt provides possible means to circumvent blockade of any single step such as mTOR.

Targeting translocation/fusion gene products

Immunotherapy

Of all the solid tumors, sarcomas may be one of the best models for testing immunotherapy because, as discussed, many sarcomas have specific chromosomal translocations, generating fusion proteins characteristic of these sarcomas. The translocation fusion proteins, which may be responsible for the neoplastic process in these tumors, would be ideal targets for immunotherapy. Thus, although it becomes theoretically possible to exploit the gene fusions as novel tumor antigens for immunotherapy; practically the problem has been complex. Potential problems to overcome with this line of therapy are numerous and include insufficient amounts of fusion protein expression to allow for access to the immune system, lack of proteasomal degradation of the protein into peptides appropriate for binding to major histocompatability (MHC) class I and class II molecules, lack of T cell help triggered by peptides binding class II molecules, lack of cytotoxic T lymphocyte (CTL) stimulation due to lack of peptide binding to appropriate class I MHC molecules, low affinity binding of such translocation products to MHC molecules, and expression by tumor cells of molecules such as FasL that could induce apoptosis of CTL, all of which may protect tumor cells from immune surveillance. Techniques are being developed that result in peptides derived from these fusion proteins (in conjunction with major histocompatability complex class I molecules) being expressed on the tumor cell surface so as to increase immune recognition of tumor cells. This strategy is currently being explored in sarcoma subtypes with specific translocations (reviewed in [87]).

Transcriptional modulation

The function of these novel fusion proteins as potent transcription factors may also be exploited to increase the delivery of cytotoxin directed treatments. Because some of the fusion transcripts have been shown to be more potent transcriptional activators than their wild-type counterparts [55], the delivery of exogenous toxic genes under the control of these regulatory elements is a potentially specific mechanism to target these tumors. Although normal cells may express the wild-type gene, its reduced transcriptional activity is proposed to result in little or no activation of the exogenous toxin. This approach been tested in alveolar rhabdomyosarcoma in which targeted expression of the diphtheria toxin A gene has resulted in expression and appropriately selective toxicity [88].

Fusion product down-regulation

The role of the EWS-FLI1 fusion gene is the pathogenesis of Ewing sarcoma was discussed earlier. Inhibition of the expression of this fusion leads to inhibition of cellular proliferation [68] through one of several purported mechanisms. Currently, small inhibitory ribonucleic acid (siRNA) is becoming a powerful and specific tool for suppressing gene expression in mammalian cells. Using siRNA technology the EWS-Fli fusion gene has been suppressed in Ewing sarcoma cell lines with dramatic effects on proliferative capacity [89]. These results represent the first application of exogenous siRNAs targeted against an endogenous tumor-specific transcript and could well lead to a new avenue of therapeutics.

Selected specific examples

Liposarcomas

Although the heterogeneity of liposarcomas makes them a difficult entity on which to perform clinical studies, the presence of multiple molecular abnormalities also provides numerous rationale targets for therapeutic intervention. For example, the antidiabetic thiazoladinedione drug family binds to the receptor PPAR-gamma. This receptor is present on the cell surface of many liposarcomas. When PPAR-gamma engages its ligand, it induces differentiation of the liposarcoma cell toward an adipocyte, with abundant fat droplet accumulation and decreased S-phase fraction. This laboratory finding has led to several ongoing trials of these drugs patients with advanced liposarcoma [90,91]. Also as discussed earlier, liposarcomas overexpress CDK4 (which leads to predominance of hyperphosphorylated pRb and a hyperproliferative state). Thus it makes sense that drugs that could block CDK4 activity might prove effective in the treatment of liposarcomas. One such drug is flavopiridol, a small molecule cyclin-dependent kinase inhibitor that has shown efficacy in preclinical studies and is currently in clinical trials [92].

Imatinib mesylate

No current review of this subject is complete without discussion of imatinib (reviewed extensively in [93]). The importance of the c-kit pathway for transformation in GIST was discussed earlier. Imatinib is a 2-phenylpyrimidine derivative that was rationally designed to block the binding of adenosine triphosphate to the ABL kinase [94]. Subsequent studies demonstrated that the *BCR-ABL* fusion gene product of the Philadelphia chromosome was effectively inhibited by imatinib [95]. Subsequently, more than 85% of chronic-phase CML patients achieve a complete hematologic response with imatinib [96]. However, further studies demonstrated that imatinib is not entirely specific for ABL and has significant inhibitory activity against related tyrosine kinases: PDGFRA, PDGFRB, ARG (ABL-related kinase), and KIT [97].

Two critical observations suggested that imatinib might be effective against GISTs. For one, imatinib could block the in vitro kinase activity of both wild-type KIT and a mutant KIT commonly found in GISTs. Secondly, imatinib inhibited the growth of a GIST cell line containing a *KIT* gene mutation [98]. These observations led to the compassionate use of imatinib for a patient with GIST and known metastasis to the liver. Imatinib was well tolerated in this patient, and all cancer-related symptoms disappeared. This success led to a multicenter trial and within 6 months, partial responses were observed in 54% of patients, and an additional 28% had stable disease [99]. On the basis of these results as well as the European Organization for Research and Treatment of Cancer trial, imatinib was approved by the US Food and Drug Administration for the treatment of unresectable and metastatic GIST on February 1, 2002. The phenomenal success of imatinib in a previously all but untreatable disease often obscures the fact that 14% of patients with GIST overtly progress on imatinib and that immunohistochemical studies from a number of different groups indicate that a subset of GISTs (variably estimated at 2% to 10%) have little or no KIT expression [100], highlighting the heterogeneity of this previously homogeneous entity. Furthermore, loss of KIT expression is observed in some advanced GISTs that have become imatinib resistant. Preliminary studies of GISTs have identified four mechanisms for imatinib resistance: (1) acquisition of a secondary point mutation in *KIT* resulting in imatinib resistance (approximately 90% of KIT-low/negative patients will have either a secondary mutation in KIT or a mutation in platelet-derived growth factor receptor [PDGFR]); (2) enhanced KIT kinase activity secondary to genomic amplification; (3) compensation for KIT loss by up-regulation of as of yet unidentified tyrosine kinase, perhaps src based on success of a src-specific drug in imatinib-resistant CML [101,102]; and (4) in vivo resistance due to unidentified "extrinsic factors" not observed in vitro [103]. However, with imatinib as a model, several multi-targeted tyrosine kinase inhibitors are in clinical trials with early promising results.

Summary

Great insights into the molecular mechanisms that lead to the formation of sarcomas have been gained over the last decade. The fusion products inherent to certain subtypes of sarcomas have been cloned, and their mechanisms of action are currently being elucidated. Similarly, much progress has been made in the understanding of signal transduction cascades that are dysregulated in sarcomas. In both these cases advancements are already contributing to clinical practice. However, much more remains to be learned for the translocation-specific sarcomas, and those with identifiable signal transduction cascade abnormalities make up only a small percentage of the 10,000 patients with newly diagnosed sarcomas presenting for recommendations for treatment options in the United States annually. It is hoped that as the molecular targets are better elucidated that more people with a variety of sarcomas will have the benefit observed with imatinib in patients with GIST and dermatofibrosarcoma protuberans.

Most notably absent from this review is any discussion of leiomyosarcoma (LMS) and malignant fibrous histiocytoma (MFH, now termed "undifferentiated high grade pleomorphic sarcoma" in the latest fascicle from the World Health Organization), as well as osteogenic sarcoma and conventional chondrosarcoma, two of the most common sarcomas of soft tissue and bone, respectively. The lack of discussion about these sarcoma subtypes is a reflection on our current understanding of their biology. As a case in point, LMS includes uterine LMS (often grouped under "uterine cancer"), as well as LMS that arise in the retroperitoneum or extremity. All are pathologically indistinguishable, yet they have distinct clinical behaviors and respond differently to chemotherapy. The molecular basis for these distinctions is unclear. In LMS, it is believed that differentiating smooth muscle cells are the precursors, whereas in the case of MFH even the precursor cells are unknown.

In conclusion, although many more details remain to be elucidated, the hope is that the knowledge that has been obtained from the study of better characterized sarcomas will be applicable to more common aneuploid sarcomas, as well as to solid tumors as a whole. Progress at the laboratory bench in this rare and unusual group of cancers will result in an acceleration of treatments for these and more common cancers at the patient's bedside.

References

[1] Cormier JN, Pollock RE. Soft tissue sarcomas. CA Cancer J Clin 2004;54(2):94–109.

[2] Singh HK, Kilpatrick SE, Silverman JF. Fine needle aspiration biopsy of soft tissue sarcomas: utility and diagnostic challenges. Adv Anat Pathol 2004;11(1):24–37.

[3] Fletcher JA. Molecular biology and cytogenetics of soft tissue sarcomas: relevance for targeted therapies. Cancer Treat Res 2004;120:99–116.

[4] Khan J, Wei JS, Ringner M, et al. Classification and diagnostic prediction of cancers using gene expression profiling and artificial neural networks. Nat Med 2001;7(6):673–9.

[5] Oliveira AM, Fletcher CD. Molecular prognostication for soft tissue sarcomas: are we ready yet? J Clin Oncol 2004;22(20):4031–4.

[6] Jemal A, Tiwari RC, Murray T, et al. Cancer statistics, 2004. CA Cancer J Clin 2004;54(1):8–29.

[7] Orlow I, Drobnjak M, Zhang ZF, et al. Alterations of INK4A and INK4B genes in adult soft tissue sarcomas: effect on survival. J Natl Cancer Inst 1999;91(1):73–9.

[8] Mertens F, Stromberg U, Mandahl N, et al. Prognostically important chromosomal aberrations in soft tissue sarcomas: a report of the Chromosomes and Morphology (CHAMP) Study Group. Cancer Res 2002;62(14):3980–4.

[9] Kawaguchi K, Oda Y, Saito T, et al. Mechanisms of inactivation of the p16INK4a gene in leiomyosarcoma of soft tissue: decreased p16 expression correlates with promoter methylation and poor prognosis. J Pathol 2003;201(3):487–95.

[10] Segal NH, Pavlidis P, Antonescu CR, et al. Classification and subtype prediction of adult soft tissue sarcoma by functional genomics. Am J Pathol 2003;163(2):691–700.

[11] Knezevich SR, Garnett MJ, Pysher TJ, et al. ETV6-NTRK3 gene fusions and trisomy 11 establish a histogenetic link between mesoblastic nephroma and congenital fibrosarcoma. Cancer Res 1998;58(22):5046–8.
[12] Baker SJ, Kinzler KW, Vogelstein B. Knudson's hypothesis and the TP53 revolution. Genes Chromosomes Cancer 2003;38(4):329.
[13] Oda Y, Sakamoto A, Saito T, et al. Expression of hepatocyte growth factor (HGF)/scatter factor and its receptor c-MET correlates with poor prognosis in synovial sarcoma. Hum Pathol 2000; 31(2):185–92.
[14] Fligman I, Lonardo F, Jhanwar SC, et al. Molecular diagnosis of synovial sarcoma and characterization of a variant SYT-SSX2 fusion transcript. Am J Pathol 1995;147(6):1592–9.
[15] Seol DW, Zarnegar R. Structural and functional characterization of the mouse c-met proto-oncogene (hepatocyte growth factor receptor) promoter. Biochim Biophys Acta 1998;1395(3): 252–8.
[16] Fresno Vara JA, Casado E, de Castro J, et al. PI3K/Akt signalling pathway and cancer. Cancer Treat Rev 2004;30(2):193–204.
[17] Abramson DH, Frank CM. Second nonocular tumors in survivors of bilateral retinoblastoma: a possible age effect on radiation-related risk. Ophthalmology 1998;105(4):573–9 [discussion: 579–80].
[18] Wong FL, Boice Jr JD, Abramson DH, et al. Cancer incidence after retinoblastoma. Radiation dose and sarcoma risk. JAMA 1997;278(15):1262–7.
[19] Sherr CJ, McCormick F. The RB and p53 pathways in cancer. Cancer Cell 2002;2(2):103–12.
[20] Macleod K. Tumor suppressor genes. Curr Opin Genet Dev 2000;10(1):81–93.
[21] Kim SH, Cho NH, Tallini G, et al. Prognostic role of cyclin D1 in retroperitoneal sarcomas. Cancer 2001;91(2):428–34.
[22] Wei G, Lonardo F, Ueda T, et al. CDK4 gene amplification in osteosarcoma: reciprocal relationship with INK4A gene alterations and mapping of 12q13 amplicons. Int J Cancer 1999;80(2):199–204.
[23] Sigal A, Rotter V. Oncogenic mutations of the p53 tumor suppressor: the demons of the guardian of the genome. Cancer Res 2000;60(24):6788–93.
[24] Creager AJ, Cohen JA, Geradts J. Aberrant expression of cell-cycle regulatory proteins in human mesenchymal neoplasia. Cancer Detect Prev 2001;25(2):123–31.
[25] Wang S, El-Deiry WS. The p53 pathway: targets for the development of novel cancer therapeutics. Cancer Treat Res 2004;119:175–87.
[26] Fingerman IM, Briggs SD. p53-mediated transcriptional activation: from test tube to cell. Cell 2004;117(6):690–1.
[27] Regula KM, Kirshenbaum LA. p53 activates the mitochondrial death pathway and apoptosis of ventricular myocytes independent of de novo gene transcription. J Mol Cell Cardiol 2001; 33(8):1435–45.
[28] Leach FS, Tokino T, Meltzer P, et al. p53 Mutation and MDM2 amplification in human soft tissue sarcomas. Cancer Res 1993;53(10 Suppl):2231–4.
[29] Oda Y, Sakamoto A, Saito T, et al. Molecular abnormalities of p53, MDM2, and H-ras in synovial sarcoma. Mod Pathol 2000;13(9):994–1004.
[30] Hieken TJ, Das Gupta TK. Mutant p53 expression: a marker of diminished survival in well-differentiated soft tissue sarcoma. Clin Cancer Res 1996;2(8):1391–5.
[31] Kawai A, Noguchi M, Beppu Y, et al. Nuclear immunoreaction of p53 protein in soft tissue sarcomas. A possible prognostic factor. Cancer 1994;73(10):2499–505.
[32] Li FP, Fraumeni Jr JF. Rhabdomyosarcoma in children: epidemiologic study and identification of a familial cancer syndrome. J Natl Cancer Inst 1969;43(6):1365–73.
[33] Shing DC, McMullan DJ, Roberts P, et al. FUS/ERG gene fusions in Ewing's tumors. Cancer Res 2003;63(15):4568–76.
[34] Rubin BP, Schuetze SM, Eary JF, et al. Molecular targeting of platelet-derived growth factor B by imatinib mesylate in a patient with metastatic dermatofibrosarcoma protuberans. J Clin Oncol 2002;20(17):3586–91.

[35] Brisset S, Schleiermacher G, Peter M, et al. CGH analysis of secondary genetic changes in Ewing tumors: correlation with metastatic disease in a series of 43 cases. Cancer Genet Cytogenet 2001;130(1):57–61.
[36] Albertson DG, Collins C, McCormick F, et al. Chromosome aberrations in solid tumors. Nat Genet 2003;34(4):369–76.
[37] Jallepalli PV, Lengauer C. Chromosome segregation and cancer: cutting through the mystery. Nat Rev Cancer 2001;1(2):109–17.
[38] Cahill DP, Lengauer C, Yu J, et al. Mutations of mitotic checkpoint genes in human cancers. Nature 1998;392(6673):300–3.
[39] Boveri T, editor. Zur Frage der Entstehung maligner Tumoren. Jena (Germany): Gustav Fischer Verlag; 1914 [in German].
[40] Li R, Sonik A, Stindl R, et al. Aneuploidy vs. gene mutation hypothesis of cancer: recent study claims mutation but is found to support aneuploidy. Proc Natl Acad Sci USA 2000; 97(7):3236–41.
[41] Marx J. Debate surges over the origins of genomic defects in cancer. Science 2002; 297(5581):544–6.
[42] Ulaner GA, Hoffman AR, Otero J, et al. Divergent patterns of telomere maintenance mechanisms among human sarcomas: sharply contrasting prevalence of the alternative lengthening of telomeres mechanism in Ewing's sarcomas and osteosarcomas. Genes Chromosomes Cancer 2004;41(2):155–62.
[43] Maser RS, DePinho RA. Connecting chromosomes, crisis, and cancer. Science 2002; 297(5581):565–9.
[44] Barr FG. Translocations, cancer and the puzzle of specificity. Nat Genet 1998;19(2):121–4.
[45] Dei Tos AP. Liposarcoma: new entities and evolving concepts. Ann Diagn Pathol 2000; 4(4):252–66.
[46] Wolf M, Aaltonen LA, Szymanska J, et al. Complexity of 12q13–22 amplicon in liposarcoma: microsatellite repeat analysis. Genes Chromosomes Cancer 1997;18(1):66–70.
[47] Hostein I, Pelmus M, Aurias A, et al. Evaluation of MDM2 and CDK4 amplification by real-time PCR on paraffin wax-embedded material: a potential tool for the diagnosis of atypical lipomatous tumours/well-differentiated liposarcomas. J Pathol 2004;202(1):95–102.
[48] Chene P. Inhibiting the p53–MDM2 interaction: an important target for cancer therapy. Nat Rev Cancer 2003;3(2):102–9.
[49] Pentimalli F, Dentice M, Fedele M, et al. Suppression of HMGA2 protein synthesis could be a tool for the therapy of well differentiated liposarcomas overexpressing HMGA2. Cancer Res 2003;63(21):7423–7.
[50] Fritz B, Schubert F, Wrobel G, et al. Microarray-based copy number and expression profiling in dedifferentiated and pleomorphic liposarcoma. Cancer Res 2002;62(11):2993–8.
[51] Orvieto E, Furlanetto A, Laurino L, et al. Myxoid and round cell liposarcoma: a spectrum of myxoid adipocytic neoplasia. Semin Diagn Pathol 2001;18(4):267–73.
[52] Rabbitts TH, Forster A, Larson R, et al. Fusion of the dominant negative transcription regulator CHOP with a novel gene FUS by translocation t(12;16) in malignant liposarcoma. Nat Genet 1993;4(2):175–80.
[53] Crozat A, Aman P, Mandahl N, et al. Fusion of CHOP to a novel RNA-binding protein in human myxoid liposarcoma. Nature 1993;363(6430):640–4.
[54] Schwarzbach MH, Koesters R, Germann A, et al. Comparable transforming capacities and differential gene expression patterns of variant FUS/CHOP fusion transcripts derived from soft tissue liposarcomas. Oncogene 2004;23(40):6798–805.
[55] Kuroda M, Wang X, Sok J, et al. Induction of a secreted protein by the myxoid liposarcoma oncogene. Proc Natl Acad Sci USA 1999;96(9):5025–30.
[56] Lo AW, Liao GC, Rocchi M, et al. Extreme reduction of chromosome-specific alpha-satellite array is unusually common in human chromosome 21. Genome Res 1999;9(10):895–908.
[57] Sirvent N, Forus A, Lescaut W, et al. Characterization of centromere alterations in liposarcomas. Genes Chromosomes Cancer 2000;29(2):117–29.

[58] Karpen GH, Allshire RC. The case for epigenetic effects on centromere identity and function. Trends Genet 1997;13(12):489–96.

[59] Wexler LH, Helman LJ. Pediatric soft tissue sarcomas. CA Cancer J Clin 1994;44(4):211–47.

[60] Shapiro DN, Valentine MB, Sublett JE, et al. Chromosomal sublocalization of the 2;13 translocation breakpoint in alveolar rhabdomyosarcoma. Genes Chromosomes Cancer 1992;4(3): 241–9.

[61] Chi N, Epstein JA. Getting your Pax straight: Pax proteins in development and disease. Trends Genet 2002;18(1):41–7.

[62] Kops GJ, Burgering BM. Forkhead transcription factors: new insights into protein kinase B (c-akt) signaling. J Mol Med 1999;77(9):656–65.

[63] Xia SJ, Barr FG. Analysis of the transforming and growth suppressive activities of the PAX3-FKHR oncoprotein. Oncogene 2004;23(41):6864–71.

[64] Wang W, Kumar P, Epstein J, et al. Insulin-like growth factor II and PAX3-FKHR cooperate in the oncogenesis of rhabdomyosarcoma. Cancer Res 1998;58(19):4426–33.

[65] Meyers PA, Levy AS. Ewing's sarcoma. Curr Treat Options Oncol 2000;1(3):247–57.

[66] Bhagirath T, Abe S, Nojima T, et al. Molecular analysis of a t(11;22) translocation junction in a case of Ewing's sarcoma. Genes Chromosomes Cancer 1995;13(2):126–32.

[67] May WA, Lessnick SL, Braun BS, et al. The Ewing's sarcoma EWS/FLI-1 fusion gene encodes a more potent transcriptional activator and is a more powerful transforming gene than FLI-1. Mol Cell Biol 1993;13(12):7393–8.

[68] Arvand A, Welford SM, Teitell MA, et al. The COOH-terminal domain of FLI-1 is necessary for full tumorigenesis and transcriptional modulation by EWS/FLI-1. Cancer Res 2001;61(13): 5311–7.

[69] Eliazer S, Spencer J, Ye D, et al. Alteration of mesodermal cell differentiation by EWS/FLI-1, the oncogene implicated in Ewing's sarcoma. Mol Cell Biol 2003;23(2):482–92.

[70] Rorie CJ, Weissman BE. The Ews/Fli-1 fusion gene changes the status of p53 in neuroblastoma tumor cell lines. Cancer Res 2004;64(20):7288–95.

[71] Ramakrishnan R, Fujimura Y, Zou JP, et al. Role of protein-protein interactions in the antiapoptotic function of EWS-Fli-1. Oncogene 2004;23(42):7087–94.

[72] Goodman RH, Smolik S. CBP/p300 in cell growth, transformation, and development. Genes Dev 2000;14(13):1553–77.

[73] Lessnick SL, Dacwag CS, Golub TR. The Ewing's sarcoma oncoprotein EWS/FLI induces a p53-dependent growth arrest in primary human fibroblasts. Cancer Cell 2002;1(4):393–401.

[74] Nakahara M, Isozaki K, Hirota S, et al. A novel gain-of-function mutation of c-kit gene in gastrointestinal stromal tumors. Gastroenterology 1998;115(5):1090–5.

[75] Rubin BP, Singer S, Tsao C, et al. KIT activation is a ubiquitous feature of gastrointestinal stromal tumors. Cancer Res 2001;61(22):8118–21.

[76] Sircar K, Hewlett BR, Huizinga JD, et al. Interstitial cells of Cajal as precursors of gastrointestinal stromal tumors. Am J Surg Pathol 1999;23(4):377–89.

[77] Hirota S, Isozaki K, Nishida T, et al. Effects of loss-of-function and gain-of-function mutations of c-kit on the gastrointestinal tract. J Gastroenterol 2000;35(Suppl 12):75–9.

[78] Williams DE, Eisenman J, Baird A, et al. Identification of a ligand for the c-kit proto-oncogene. Cell 1990;63(1):167–74.

[79] Sattler M, Salgia R. Targeting c-Kit mutations: basic science to novel therapies. Leuk Res 2004;28(Suppl 1):S11–20.

[80] Hay N, Sonenberg N. Upstream and downstream of mTOR. Genes Dev 2004;18(16):1926–45.

[81] Mitsiades CS, Mitsiades N, Koutsilieris M. The Akt pathway: molecular targets for anti-cancer drug development. Curr Cancer Drug Targets 2004;4(3):235–56.

[82] Longobardi L, Torello M, Buckway C, et al. A novel insulin-like growth factor (IGF)-independent role for IGF binding protein-3 in mesenchymal chondroprogenitor cell apoptosis. Endocrinology 2003;144(5):1695–702.

[83] Scavo LM, Karas M, Murray M, et al. Insulin-like growth factor-I stimulates both cell growth and lipogenesis during differentiation of human mesenchymal stem cells into adipocytes. J Clin Endocrinol Metab 2004;89(7):3543–53.

[84] Strammiello R, Benini S, Manara MC, et al. Impact of IGF-I/IGF-IR circuit on the angiogenetic properties of Ewing's sarcoma cells. Horm Metab Res 2003;35(11–12):675–84.
[85] Xie Y, Skytting B, Nilsson G, et al. Expression of insulin-like growth factor-1 receptor in synovial sarcoma: association with an aggressive phenotype. Cancer Res 1999;59(15): 3588–91.
[86] Gallicchio MA, van Sinderen M, Bach LA. Insulin-like growth factor binding protein-6 and CCI-779, an ester analogue of rapamycin, additively inhibit rhabdomyosarcoma growth. Horm Metab Res 2003;35(11–12):822–7.
[87] Maki RG. Immunity against soft-tissue sarcomas. Curr Oncol Rep 2003;5(4):282–7.
[88] Massuda ES, Dunphy EJ, Redman RA, et al. Regulated expression of the diphtheria toxin A chain by a tumor-specific chimeric transcription factor results in selective toxicity for alveolar rhabdomyosarcoma cells. Proc Natl Acad Sci USA 1997;94(26):14701–6.
[89] Chansky HA, Barahmand-Pour F, Mei Q, et al. Targeting of EWS/FLI-1 by RNA interference attenuates the tumor phenotype of Ewing's sarcoma cells in vitro. J Orthop Res 2004;22(4): 910–7.
[90] Debrock G, Vanhentenrijk V, Sciot R, et al. A phase II trial with rosiglitazone in liposarcoma patients. Br J Cancer 2003;89(8):1409–12.
[91] Gauthier A, Vassiliou G, Benoist F, et al. Adipocyte low density lipoprotein receptor-related protein gene expression and function is regulated by peroxisome proliferator-activated receptor gamma. J Biol Chem 2003;278(14):11945–53.
[92] Senderowicz AM. Small molecule modulators of cyclin-dependent kinases for cancer therapy. Oncogene 2000;19(56):6600–6.
[93] Ross DM, Hughes TP. Cancer treatment with kinase inhibitors: what have we learnt from imatinib? Br J Cancer 2004;90(1):12–9.
[94] Buchdunger E, Zimmermann J, Mett H, et al. Inhibition of the Abl protein-tyrosine kinase in vitro and in vivo by a 2-phenylaminopyrimidine derivative. Cancer Res 1996;56(1):100–4.
[95] Druker BJ, Tamura S, Buchdunger E, et al. Effects of a selective inhibitor of the Abl tyrosine kinase on the growth of Bcr-Abl positive cells. Nat Med 1996;2(5):561–6.
[96] Deininger MW, O'Brien SG, Ford JM, et al. Practical management of patients with chronic myeloid leukemia receiving imatinib. J Clin Oncol 2003;21(8):1637–47.
[97] Pardanani A, Tefferi A. Imatinib targets other than bcr/abl and their clinical relevance in myeloid disorders. Blood 2004;104(7):1931–9.
[98] Tuveson DA, Willis NA, Jacks T, et al. STI571 inactivation of the gastrointestinal stromal tumor c-KIT oncoprotein: biological and clinical implications. Oncogene 2001;20(36):5054–8.
[99] Dagher R, Cohen M, Williams G, et al. Approval summary: imatinib mesylate in the treatment of metastatic and/or unresectable malignant gastrointestinal stromal tumors. Clin Cancer Res 2002;8(10):3034–8.
[100] Medeiros F, Corless CL, Duensing A, et al. KIT-negative gastrointestinal stromal tumors: proof of concept and therapeutic implications. Am J Surg Pathol 2004;28(7):889–94.
[101] Golas JM, Arndt K, Etienne C, et al. SKI-606, a 4-anilino-3-quinolinecarbonitrile dual inhibitor of Src and Abl kinases, is a potent antiproliferative agent against chronic myelogenous leukemia cells in culture and causes regression of K562 xenografts in nude mice. Cancer Res 2003;63(2):375–81.
[102] Shah NP, Tran C, Lee FY, et al. Overriding imatinib resistance with a novel ABL kinase inhibitor [comment]. Science 2004;305(5682):399–401.
[103] Duensing A, Medeiros F, McConarty B, et al. Mechanisms of oncogenic KIT signal transduction in primary gastrointestinal stromal tumors (GISTs). Oncogene 2004;23(22):3999–4006.

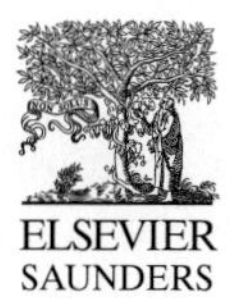

ELSEVIER
SAUNDERS

Hematol Oncol Clin N Am
19 (2005) 451–470

HEMATOLOGY/
ONCOLOGY
CLINICS OF
NORTH AMERICA

Surgical Management of Sarcomas

Edward Y. Cheng, MD[a,b,*]

[a]*Department of Orthopaedic Surgery, University of Minnesota, 2512 South 7th Street, R200, Minneapolis, MN 55454, USA*
[b]*Orthopaedic Surgery Service, Fairview-University Medical Center, 2450 Riverside Avenue South, Minneapolis, MN 55454, USA*

The treatment of sarcomas has become multidisciplinary, as advances in biology, imaging, chemotherapy, and radiation have improved the outlook for patients who have these cancers. Surgery, however, remains the mainstay of treatment as the management of nearly all tumors will encompass surgical considerations. Whether for diagnostic, staging, tumor excision, or palliative indications, it is essential that the evaluation be performed early and by a surgeon who is routinely familiar with all aspects of sarcoma treatment, lest any mismanagement complicate or preclude treatment options later in the patient's course of disease.

Clinical presentation and physical examination

Frequently the patient who has a bone or soft tissue sarcoma will present initially to a surgeon after a mass is either discovered by self-examination or unmasked by imaging studies obtained because of an injury or even pathologic fracture. On careful questioning, many patients will admit to a prodromal course of pain or aching discomfort, although painless masses are also common. The presence of radicular symptoms or a Tinel's sign may be caused by peripheral

* Department of Orthopaedic Surgery, University of Minnesota, 2512 South 7th Street, R200, Minneapolis, MN 55454.

E-mail address: cheng002@umn.edu

0889-8588/05/$ – see front matter
doi:10.1016/j.hoc.2005.03.009

nerve compression or involvement with a tumor mass. Limited joint range of motion may result from the presence of a large mass in a periarticular site. Arterial occlusion is rare, even when tumor growth surrounds an arterial structure, but venous congestion may occur with large tumors. Pain during weight bearing suggests that there has been some loss of strength in the structural integrity of the underlying bone. Transillumination of masses that grow into subcutaneous locations is highly suggestive of a synovial or Baker's cyst. Associated cutaneous findings, such as the hyperpigmentation of café-au-lait spots in neurofibromatosis, raise the likelihood of a systemic disease.

Evaluation

It is preferable to complete most diagnostic evaluations before performing any type of biopsy, as the findings of these evaluations may influence either the lesion that is biopsied or the diagnostic histopathologic tests performed. The best screening study for a bone lesion is plain radiography because of its low cost, expediency, and ability to distinguish between benign and aggressive or malignant bony lesions. In addition, radiographs may be also be useful for soft tissue lesions, as findings such as calcifications are suggestive of either vascular tumors or some soft tissue sarcomas (synovial sarcoma). In contrast, MRI is valuable for providing insight into the tissue of origin (myxoid, fat, fibrous, vascular) and a "map" to assess the location, extent, and relationship to surrounding structures of bone and soft tissue masses (Fig. 1A–C); however, the MRI signal characteristics of a tumor are not as helpful in assessing the malignant potential of a mass. For most bone or soft tissue masses, the optimal imaging of the primary tumor will include both radiographs and an MRI study (Fig. 2A–C).

Staging is best done using computerized axial tomography (CAT) of the lung, as most sarcomas will spread to the lung as the first site of metastasis. Because liposarcoma has a higher incidence of extrapulmonary spread [1,2], positron emission tomography (PET) using [F-18]-fluorodeoxy-D-glucose (FDG) may be useful in this histologic subtype. Osteosarcomas may spread to the bone and therefore a technicium-99 bone scan is essential for staging. If a diagnosis of rhabdomyosarcoma is suspected, a bone marrow biopsy is used to rule out a higher stage tumor; bone marrow biopsies are often part of protocol-directed therapy for pediatric Ewing sarcoma/primitive neuroectodermal tumor (PNET). Some soft tissue sarcoma histologies (epithelioid sarcoma, rhabdomyosarcoma, clear cell sarcoma, synovial sarcoma) have a higher propensity for lymph node metastasis and so sentinel lymph node biopsy may be useful; however, the rarity of these tumors precludes the ability to validate an objective benefit [3–5]. The role of functional imaging using FDG-PET scanning is established in some cancers (lung, melanoma, lymphoma) and is currently evolving for sarcomas (see article by Schuetze elsewhere in this issue). Its greatest utility may be in

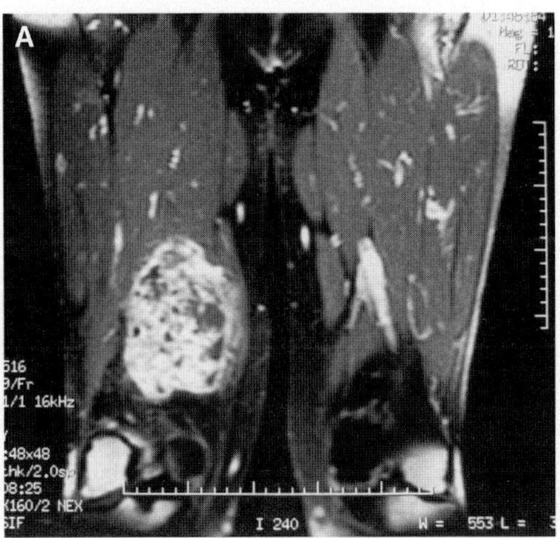

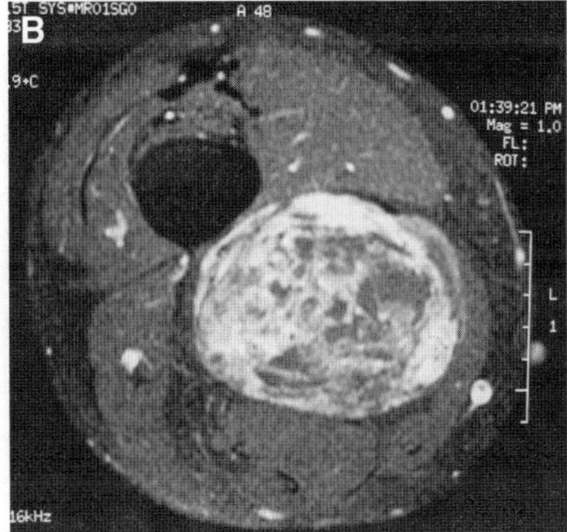

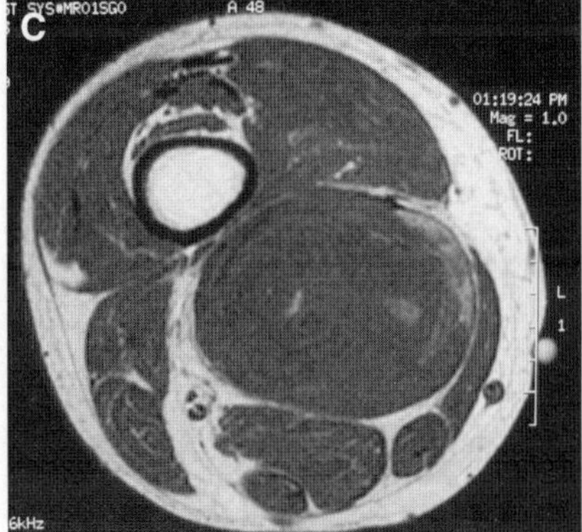

Fig. 1. (*A*) Coronal fat suppression MRI of myxoid and round cell liposarcoma of posterior thigh. (*B*) Axial fat suppression MRI of myxoid and round cell liposarcoma of posterior thigh with abutment against popliteal artery. (*C*) Axial T1-weighted MRI of same tumor.

staging, assessing a tumor's response to neoadjuvant treatment, or surveillance follow-up studies (Fig. 3) [6–9].

Biopsy

The explosion of molecular biologic advances in understanding these diseases has led to an evolving classification and an improvement in the diagnostic accuracy in sarcomas. Consequently, the biopsy of a potential sarcoma, although usually straightforward technically, involves considerable cognitive activity

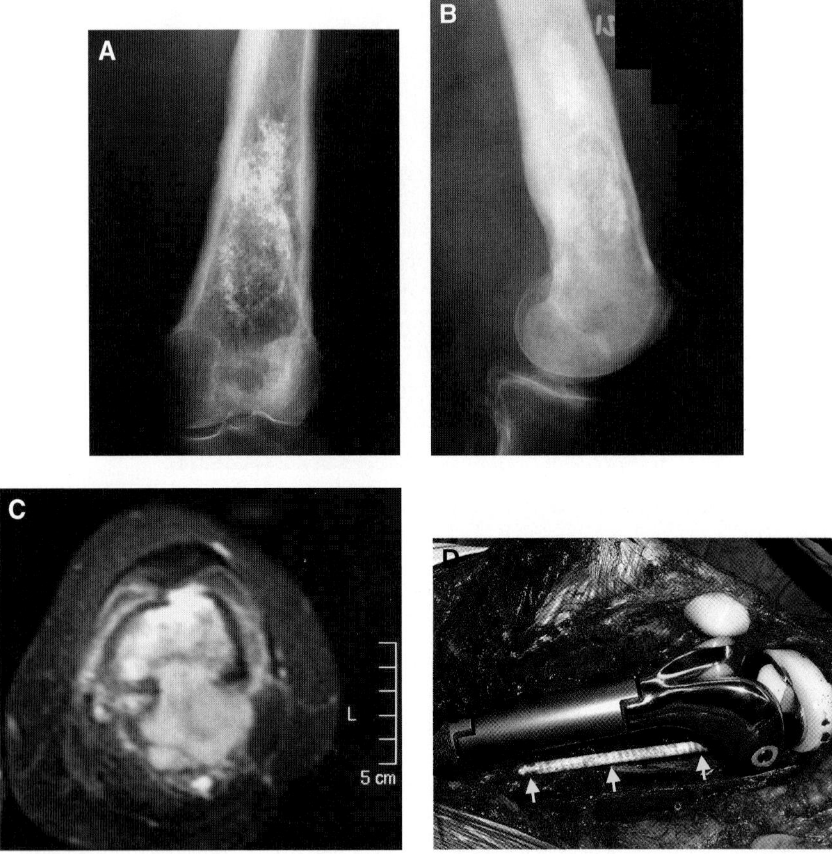

Fig. 2. Anterior-posterior (*A*) and lateral (*B*) radiographs of distal femoral chondrosarcoma. Note extraosseous extension into soft tissues. (*C*) Axial fat suppression MRI of distal femur at level of patella demonstrating large posterior soft tissue mass extension and involvement of popliteal artery and vein structures. (*D*) Intraoperative photograph of distal femoral rotating hinge knee prosthesis with associated popliteal artery interpositional arterial gortex graft (*arrows*) reconstruction. Proximal on left, distal on right, anterior on top, and posterior on bottom. Quadriceps muscle retracted anteriorly with undersurface of patellar button prosthesis shown above femoral component prosthesis.

to avoid any hazards. An ill-placed needle or incision may convert a resectable tumor into an unresectable situation requiring an amputation [10]. In addition, an improper diagnosis can lead to suboptimal treatment. Hence, if there is any concern about a mass representing a sarcoma, the biopsy should be performed by the surgeon who has experience in sarcomas and who will be managing the definitive tumor excision [11–13]. The goal of the biopsy is to provide a sufficient quantity of target tissue for diagnosis without compromising any potential therapies or subsequent surgery at a minimum of morbidity to the patient.

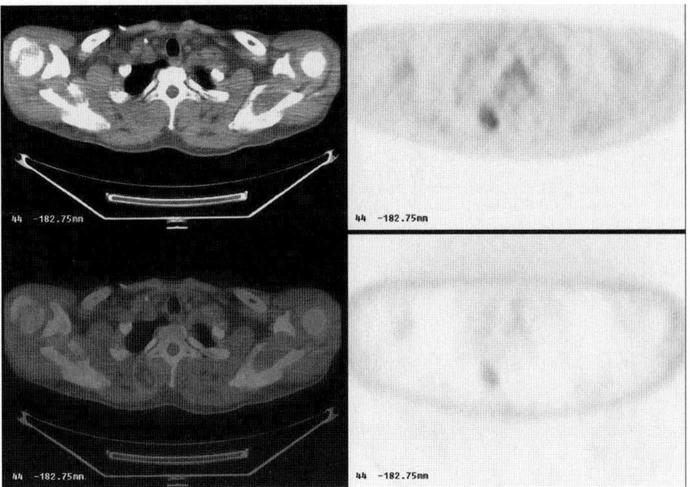

Fig. 3. CT scan (*top left*) and FDG-PET scan (*right*) and CT with PET image overlay (*bottom left*) of metastatic leiomyosarcoma to right paraspinal muscles. Tumor is highlighted orange color in CT-PET image (*bottom left*). (*See the Web version for color.*)

Excisional and incisional biopsies are acceptable techniques in specific situations. An excisional biopsy of the entire tumor mass should only be done for small, subcutaneous tumors that will leave a surgical bed that can readily be re-excised with a wide margin without undue morbidity (eg, skin grafting) should the tumor prove to be a sarcoma. Despite the cosmetic appeal of a transverse incision parallel to Langer's skin cleavage lines, transverse incisions on the extremity should never be done and longitudinal incisions should be made in extremity sites. An incisional biopsy is much safer and avoids the scenario of an inadvertent, improper removal of a sarcoma.

Incisional biopsies can be done using a percutaneous needle or open technique. The optimal technique is controversial, even among institutions experienced in sarcoma management. However, if a needle is chosen, most institutions have ceased using aspiration cytology and instead rely on a Tru-Cut (Allegiance/Cardinal Health, McGaw Park, Illinois) or similar core needle device to obtain a core sliver of tissue. An open biopsy provides a larger quantity of tissue at the expense of a surgical procedure. Contamination of surrounding tissue must be minimized and ironically is not necessarily lower with a needle technique. Hemorrhage can be recognized and controlled immediately with an open incision, whereas multiple passes with a large diameter core needle may cause significant occult oozing into the subcutaneous tissues in the ensuing 24 hours that is not recognized at the time of biopsy. Prolonged compression and immobilization of the affected body part may help mitigate this possibility when performing needle biopsies.

As the biopsy tract should be excised when the tumor itself is resected, the biopsy tract placement is of utmost importance and the incision should be made

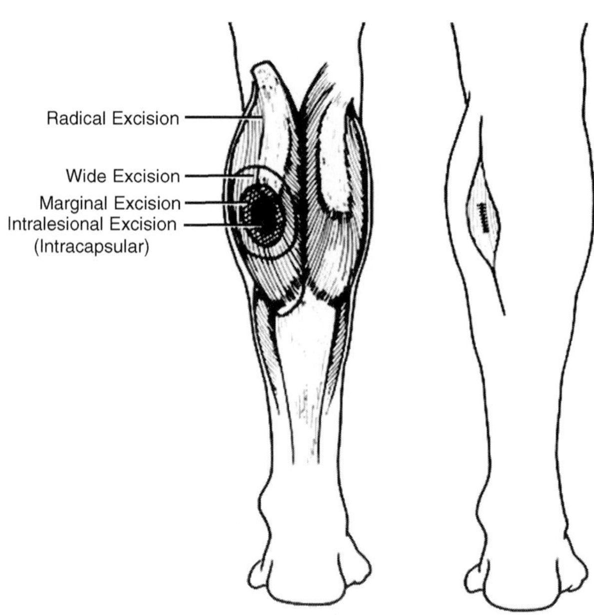

Fig. 4. Schematic drawing of soft tissue mass of gastrocnemius muscle. Surgical margins on left and surgical incision encompassing previous biopsy track on right. (*From* Cheng EY. Benign soft tissue tumors. In: Craig EV, editor. Textbook of orthopaedic surgery. Media (PA): Williams and Wilkins; 1999. p. 1006; with permission.)

in line with the subsequent extensile incision (Fig. 4). Major neurologic and vascular structures should not be exposed or contaminated and dissection should be done within muscle tissue as opposed to through known tissue planes. Palpation or MRI mapping is useful for targeting the tumor. The location within the tumor itself is also important to avoid sampling necrotic tissue. Fresh tissue should be saved for molecular studies and lymphoma markers if this diagnosis is a possibility. Optimally, tissue should be stored in a frozen tissue bank. If there is any possibility of an infectious origin to the mass, cultures should be obtained. For bone lesions, the soft tissue mass outside the bone usually provides sufficient viable tissue for diagnosis and avoids the difficulties associated with decalcification of hard bone. A frozen section at the time of biopsy is useful to ensure capture of diagnostic material and avoids erroneous biopsies.

Some anatomic sites may have special considerations. For sacral tumors, needle biopsies are associated with a higher incidence of error [14] and may result in a delay in treatment. Intra-abdominal and retroperitoneal tumors may be difficult to access and at times may require performing a core needle biopsy in a controlled setting after exposing the tumor through either traditional mini-laparotomy or laparoscopy. Similarly, tumors arising in the popliteal, groin, or deep forearm locations may be difficult to biopsy blindly with a core needle because of surrounding neurovascular structures, and therefore a small incision or CT guidance is useful.

Surgical indications

The indication for surgical excision depends on the tissue diagnosis and stage of the sarcoma. For most nonmetastatic bone and soft tissue sarcomas (excluding rhabdomyosarcoma), surgical resection of the tumor, in combination with chemotherapy or radiation, is indicated as long as the morbidity of excision is not excessive. For Ewings sarcoma family of tumors (ESFTs) located in anatomic locations difficult to address surgically without substantial morbidity, such as the spine or pelvis, resection is controversial [15] and local control using radiation instead of surgery in combination with chemotherapy has been reported [16,17]. In patients who have metastatic bone or soft tissue sarcomas, local control of the primary lesion is a goal in conjunction with overall control of the disease, and the timing and indication for surgical treatment of the primary site will depend on numerous factors best determined by a dedicated multidisciplinary sarcoma team.

Timing of surgery

Surgical excision of nonmetastatic osteosarcoma [18,19] and ESFTs can be undertaken either before or after adjuvant chemotherapy without any significant difference in survival. Most centers favor chemotherapy before excision because of the advantages of observing the tumor response to chemotherapy and likely tumor shrinkage (Fig. 5A, B) that occurs when sequencing treatment in this manner. For soft tissue sarcomas (excluding rhabdomyosarcoma), multimodal therapy differs considerably among major cancer centers; however, surgical excision is consistently performed before, during, or after chemotherapy or radiation without any major differences in survivorship [20–23].

Resectability and limb salvage surgery

Whether or not a sarcoma is considered resectable depends on the morbidity associated with removal of surrounding structures. For surgery performed with a curative intent, an en bloc excision of the tumor and biopsy tract with a negative and wide surgical margin is the goal. A poorly planned biopsy may affect the resectability of a tumor [10]. Advances in the reconstruction of colorectal, urologic, vascular, spine, long bone, and joint deficiencies have extended the boundaries of the term "resectable." Although most neurologic structures can-

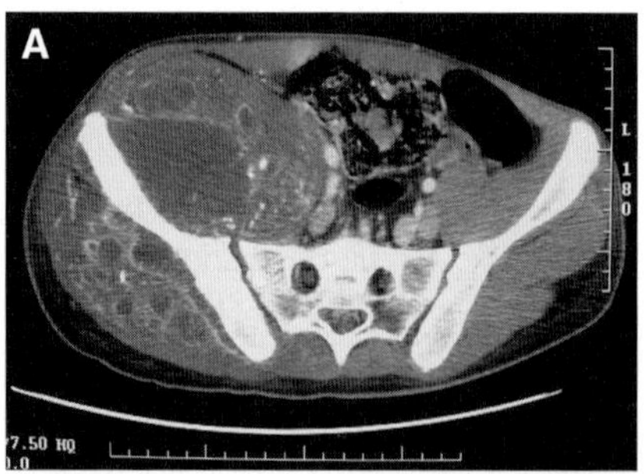

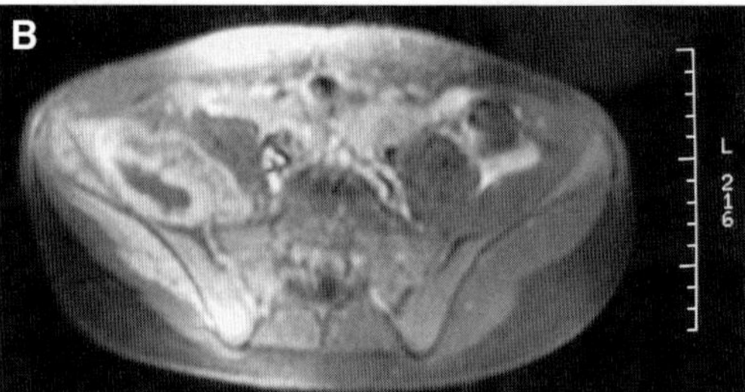

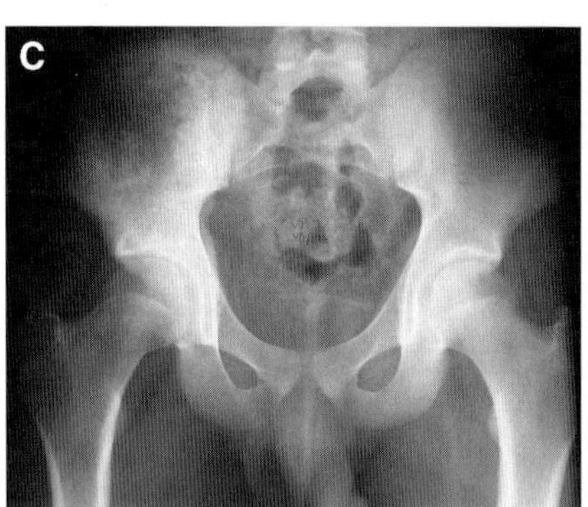

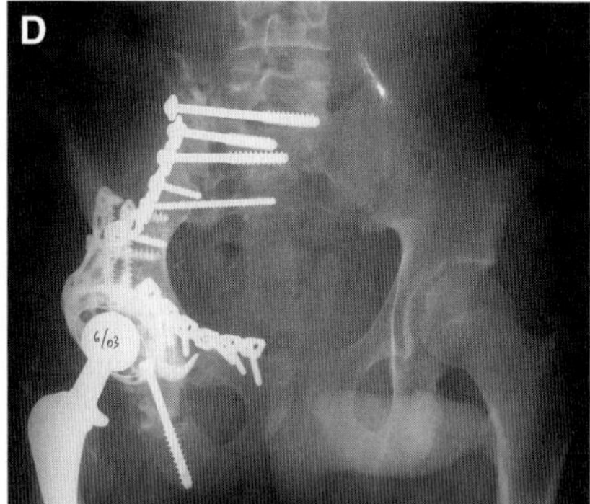

Fig. 5. (*A*) Axial CT scan of right pelvic innominate bone osteosarcoma showing large intrapelvic and extrapelvic soft tissue extension before administration of neoadjuvant chemotherapy. (*B*) Axial MRI of pelvis at same level of (*A*) demonstrating shrinkage of soft tissue mass after undergoing neoadjuvant chemotherapy for osteosarcoma. (*C*) Osteosarcoma of right pelvic innominate bone. (*D*) Anterior-posterior radiograph of pelvis demonstrating reconstruction, after modified internal hemipelvectomy, using hemipelvic allograft-prosthetic composite and total hip arthroplasty. Compression plate internal fixation of reconstructed sacroiliac joint and superior pubic ramus. Cemented total hip arthroplasty with acetabular metallic cage. (*E*) Axial CT scan demonstrating right hemipelvis allograft with posterior sacroiliac joint compression and screw fixation. (*F*) Three-dimensional CT scan reconstruction of right hemipelvis allograft reconstruction with total hip arthroplasty. (*G*) Three-dimensional CT scan reconstruction using software enhancement to contrast bone tissue against metallic hip prosthesis and internal fixation.

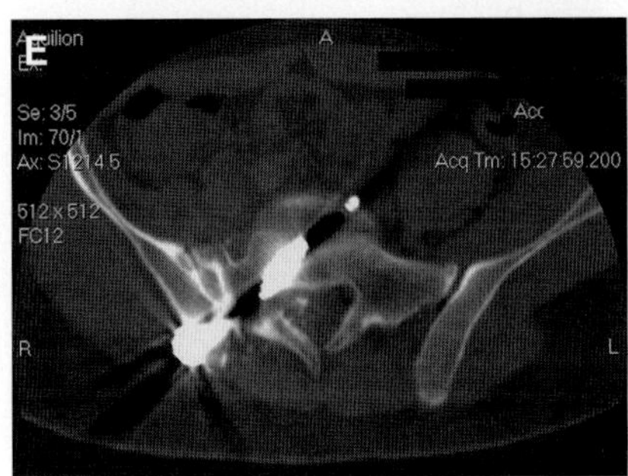

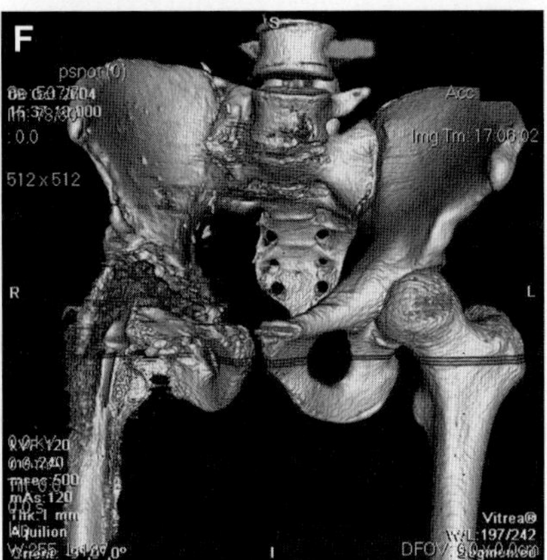

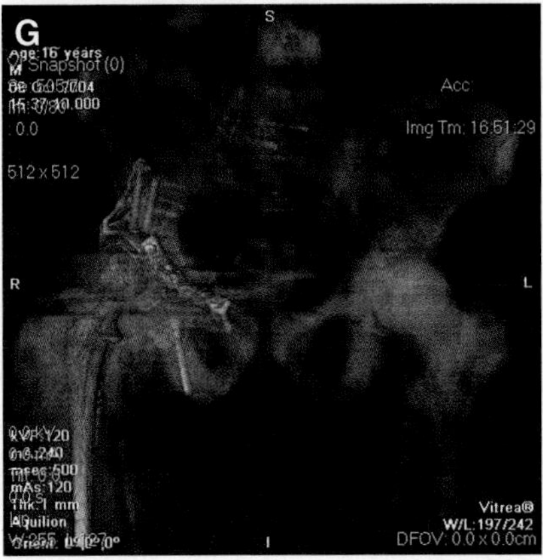

Fig. 5 (*continued*).

not be reconstructed, functional restoration after peripheral nerve deficits by performing tendon transfers does reduce the morbidity of nerve resection in specific situations. Outcomes measurement instruments have demonstrated that most patients are willing to accept major reductions in function if survivorship can be improved with surgical excision of their tumor [15].

Most bone and soft tissue sarcomas arise in the pelvis, buttock, or extremity. Limb salvage surgery can be considered as long as a reasonable reconstructive option exists after removal of the tumor. Large skeletal defects, including pelvic sarcomas (Fig. 5A–G), can be reconstructed using either large segment allografts or endoprostheses. Similarly, osteoarticular allografts (Fig. 6A, B), modular prostheses designed for oncologic usage, or a composite of allograft and prosthetic afford a reconstructive option when a hip, knee, shoulder, or elbow is affected by a sarcoma. When the knee or elbow is involved, constrained

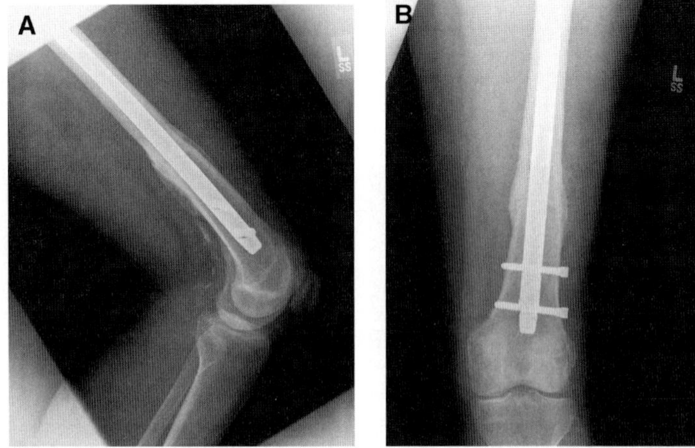

Fig. 6. Anterior-posterior (*A*) and lateral (*B*) radiographs of distal femoral osteoarticular allograft reconstruction 7 years after resection of Ewing's sarcoma.

prostheses mechanically linking both sides of the joint are necessary to maintain stability of the joint (Fig. 7A–H). Arterial reconstruction in conjunction with or without skeletal reconstruction is feasible in most cases [24–26], even in the setting of adjuvant radiation treatment (Fig. 2A–D).

The skeletally immature patient poses a unique reconstructive challenge. Functional restoration after large bony resections is achievable in most cases as long as the length of the remaining host bone is sufficient to allow fixation of an implant. The challenge is in maintaining symmetry in extremity length as the patient's contralateral extremity grows. In the past, expandable prosthesis could only be lengthened by an invasive surgery to exchange or adjust parts of the implanted device. Newer prosthetic designs with internal springs (Fig. 8A–E) or ratcheting mechanisms allow lengthening to occur by either performing a non-invasive procedure or hyper flexing the adjacent joint.

Prior excisional biopsy

At times, an excisional biopsy will have been previously performed for a presumably benign mass that turns out to be a sarcoma. Most commonly an inadvertent or unplanned excision of a sarcoma occurs with small masses. Usually there is no remaining tumor mass palpable. Nonetheless, residual tumor is present in one third of specimens re-excised after a prior unplanned excision, and several studies have demonstrated the value of re-excising the remaining tumor or surgical bed [27–30]. Optimal management should consist of a review of the prior surgeon's operative note and an MRI image of the remaining surgical tumor bed to discern the proper amount of tissue to re-excise and any possible need for a skin graft or myocutaneous flap for soft tissue closure.

Surgical margins

An adequate surgical margin is difficult to define. Certainly the plane of resection should be through nonneoplastic tissue at all times. The terms radical, wide, marginal, and intralesional (see Fig. 4) were defined for bone and soft tissue sarcomas by Enneking et al [31], but significant deficiencies exist. Al-

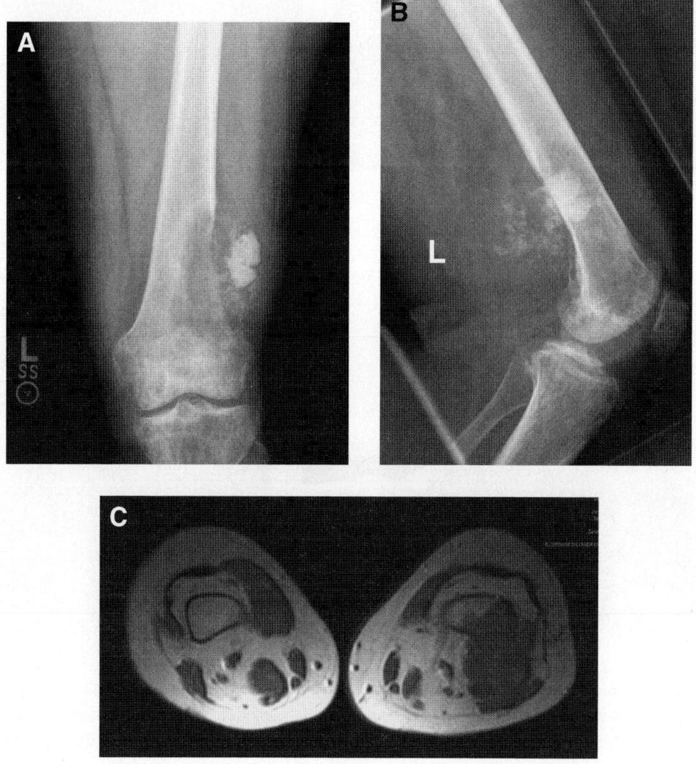

Fig. 7. (*A*) Anterior-posterior radiograph of distal femoral osteosarcoma. (*B*) Lateral radiograph of distal femoral osteosarcoma. (*C*) Axial MRI of left distal femoral osteosarcoma demonstrating soft tissue extension posterolaterally. (*D*) Coronal MRI demonstrating intramedullary extent of osteosarcoma of distal femur. (*E*) Sagittal fat suppression MRI of left distal femoral osteosarcoma demonstrating intramedullary extent of tumor and posterior soft tissue extension. (*F*) Intraoperative photograph of distal femoral replacement arthroplasty combined with rotating hinged knee prosthesis. Proximal on left, distal on right, anterior on top, and posterior on bottom. Note mechanical axial linkage between distal femoral replacement portion and plastic tibial tray prosthesis. (*G*) Anterior-posterior radiograph demonstrating appearance of distal femoral replacement prosthesis. (*H*) Lateral radiograph demonstrating same distal femoral replacement rotating hinged knee prosthesis.

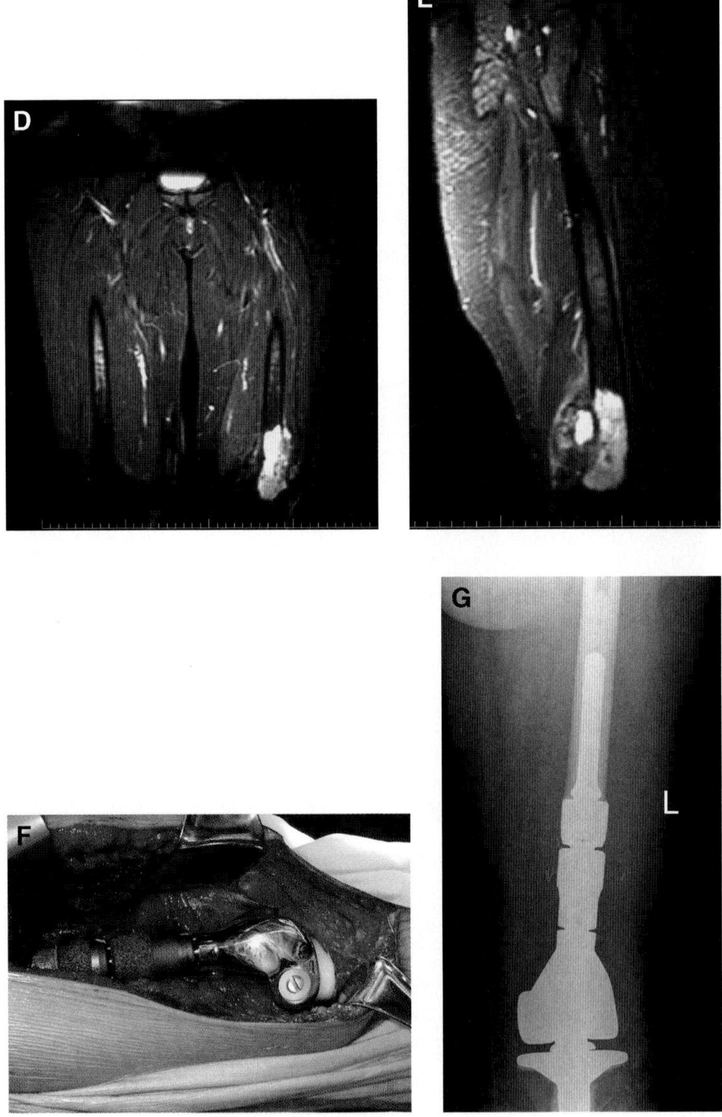

Fig. 7 (*continued*).

though ideally a wide margin outside the reactive zone of the tumor is attained, most oncologic surgeons will accept a negative but marginal margin if a plane of dissection is readily established between an important neurologic structure and the tumor mass. The surgical and pathologic analysis of surgical margins are imperfect. Surgeons may tend to overestimate the adequacy of the margin, and the retraction of muscle tissue after sectioning muscle fibers and subsequent

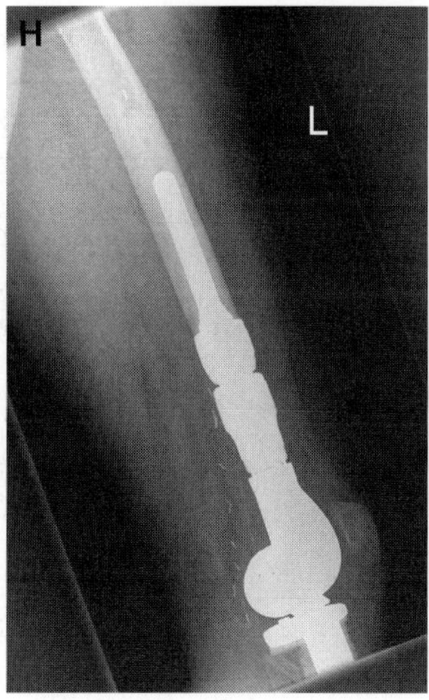

Fig. 7 (*continued*).

handling of the tumor mass may result in a pathologic analysis yielding falsely positive margins. In addition to the width of the surgical margin [32], the type of tissue at the margin is of importance. A thin 1- to 2-mm fascial barrier is much more substantial than a 1- to 2-mm margin of loose areolar or adipose tissue. There is wide agreement among oncologic surgeons, however, that a blunt plane of dissection alongside the tumor itself, so called "shell out," is inadequate and leads to a higher risk of recurrence.

Peri-operative management

There are several unique considerations to take into account when managing the surgery of a sarcoma patient. In addition to a standard preoperative assessment, additional factors to check include possible neutropenia if neoadjuvant chemotherapy was administered and examination for skin reaction or dermatitis caused by preoperative radiation. Intra-operative technical concerns include meticulous hemostasis, gentle handling of tissues to minimize necrosis, coagulation of lymphatic vessels to minimize the likelihood of lymphocele formation, fastidious wound closure, and use of myocutaneous flaps in irradiated sites or to provide soft tissue coverage over bone allografts or prostheses. Postoperative concerns are the use of long-term drains, which are frequently used beyond hospital discharge to minimize seroma formation, and temporary immobilization or limited weight-bearing of an extremity to facilitate healing balanced against the need to initiate physiotherapy and joint motion to prevent contracture. Wound healing after a sarcoma excision is compromised because the skin closure is frequently under some tension, a large soft tissue cavity and potential dead space

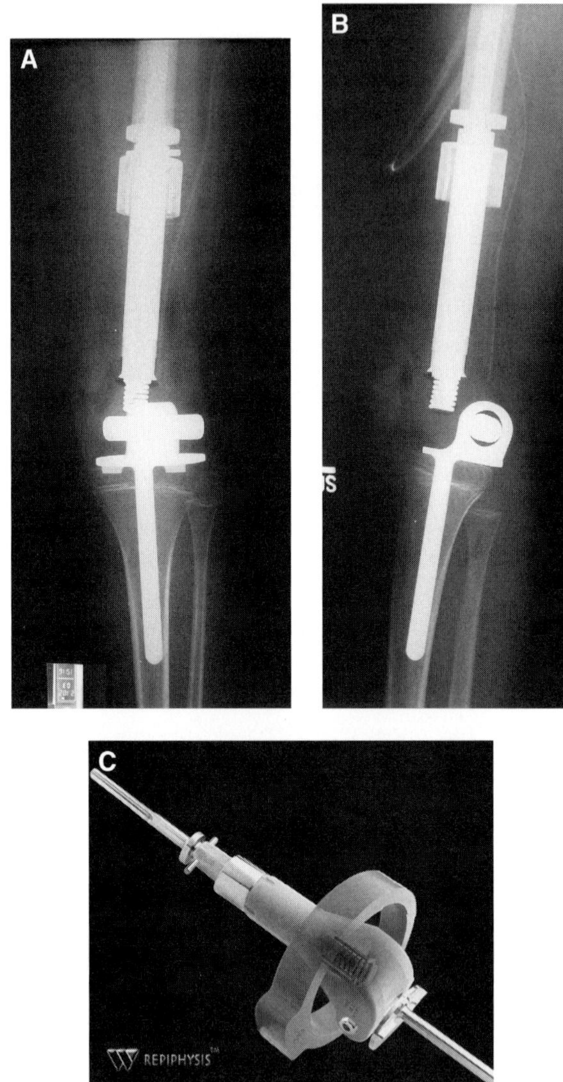

Fig. 8. (*A*) Anterior-posterior radiograph of expandable distal femoral replacement prosthesis placed in 8-year-old girl. Note placement of internal spring within radiolucent plastic housing of prosthesis. (*B*) Lateral radiograph of expandable distal femoral replacement prosthesis demonstrating internal spring within plastic polymer femoral portion. (*C*) Illustration of expandable distal femoral replacement prosthesis with internal spring highlighted. Noninvasive expansion of device is achieved using circular magnetic ring "donut" placed around patient's limb. (Courtesy of Wright Medical Technology, Inc., Arlington, TN; with permission.) Appearance of prosthesis at junction with host femur before expansion (*D*) and after activation of expansion device (*E*) demonstrating increase in length (*l*).

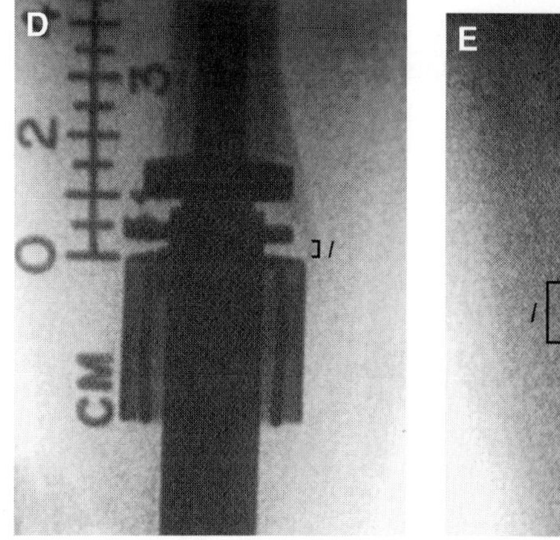

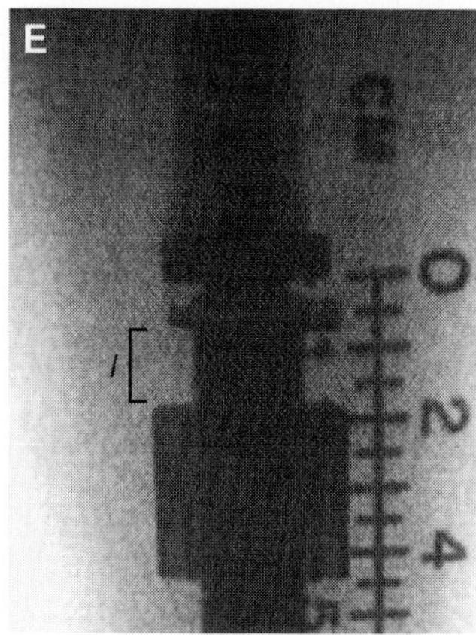

Fig. 8 (*continued*).

remains, there is poor host status caused by chemotherapy, and there is poor soft tissue status because of prior radiation. Wound infections or wound dehiscence occur in up to one third of patients receiving radiation before their tumor excision [20,33].

Oncologic outcome

Osteosarcoma and Ewing's family of tumors

The oncologic outcome after surgery and chemotherapy is undertaken for treatment of nonmetastatic osteosarcoma, and Ewing's family of tumors (EFTs) bone sarcoma has a 5-year disease-free survival (DFS) of 65% [18,19]. The main determinants of local recurrence-free survival (LRFS) and DFS are the stage of disease, site of the primary tumor, and response to induction chemotherapy.

Soft tissue sarcoma

Despite the differences in combined multimodal treatment for nonmetastatic, nonrhabdomyosarcoma soft tissue sarcomas among major sarcoma centers, the local control and disease-free survival rates after surgery are similar. For all anatomic sites combined, the 5-year DFS ranges from 65% to 75% and the 5-year LRFS ranges from 75% to 90% [20,21,34–38]. The most predictive factors for DFS and LRFS in these tumors are tumor size, grade, stage, and resection margin [39–41]. A nomogram developed at the Memorial Sloan Kettering Cancer Center based on age at diagnosis, tumor size ($\leq$5, 5–10, or >10 cm), histologic grade (high or low), histologic subtype (fibrosarcoma, leiomyosarcoma, liposarcoma, malignant fibrous histiocytoma, malignant peripheral nerve tumor, synovial, or other), depth (superficial or deep), and site (upper extremity, lower extremity, visceral, thoracic or trunk, retrointraabdominal, or head or neck) has been validated among different cancer centers for predicting DFS [42–45].

Functional outcome

Osteosarcoma and Ewing's family of tumors

The functional outcome of a bone or joint reconstruction following a sarcoma excision is highly dependent on not only the anatomic site of the primary tumor but also factors such as the extent of resection of the soft tissue muscle envelope, the type of reconstruction (ie, allograft, prosthesis, or combination of the two), and the host's baseline physical status. The Musculoskeletal Tumor Society's (MSTS) functional assessment instrument [46] is the most widely used tool for reporting results, but the Toronto Extremity Salvage Score (TESS) [47] was also adapted, validated, and proved useful. For the proximal humeral reconstruction, MSTS scores of 70% to 90% have been reported using either allograft [48] or prosthetic [49,50] reconstruction. At the distal femur, a mean MSTS score of 80 was reported for prosthetic reconstruction [51], and average MSTS function of 77% of normal has been reported [52] when using a custom prosthesis in children.

Another important parameter of success is the longevity of the reconstruction. Survivorship analysis of the reconstruction is useful for this purpose. In one of the largest series of allograft reconstructions encompassing 1100 nonpelvic massive cadaveric allografts implanted for treatment of malignant or aggressive bone tumors, 77% of the allografts remain functioning [53]. At the proximal femur, a 10-year revision free survivorship of 77% has been reported using endoprostheses. At the distal femur, a series of 110 cases of endoprosthesis reported a 93% prosthetic survivorship at 5 years and 88% at 10 years. [54]. Despite retention of either an allograft or prosthesis, re-operation is sometimes necessary for either nonunion, fracture, or wear-related failure of plastic parts of the prosthesis.

Soft tissue sarcoma

The functional outcome following surgical treatment for nonmetastatic, nonrhabdomyosarcoma soft tissue sarcomas is also highly dependent on the site and size of the primary tumor. In addition, as radiation is widely used for these tumors, wound healing complications in the short-term and radiation fibrosis in the long-term have a major impact on function [33]. The Canadian SR2 study revealed that the improvement in function postoperatively plateaus at 6 months [55]. In this trial, the mean MSTS scores at 1 year were 28 and mean TESS scores were 82. The need for major nerve resection is determined by the tumor anatomic site and extent; however, even after sciatic nerve resection for large thigh tumors

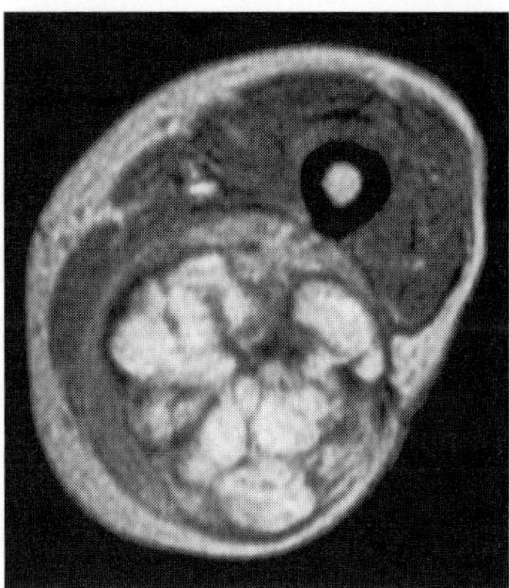

Fig. 9. Axial MRI of malignant fibrous histiocytoma surrounding sciatic nerve.

(Fig. 9), a compromised but usable extremity is salvaged and half of these patients can ambulate independently using an ankle foot orthosis [56].

Summary

Nearly all bone and soft tissue sarcomas will require surgical management. Early consultation with a surgeon who is experienced in sarcomas, before a biopsy is performed, will avoid potential errors that may complicate subsequent surgery. Advances in imaging, neoadjuvant therapies, and reconstructive techniques have improved the ability to adequately resect most bone and soft tissue sarcomas. The use of oncologic and functional outcomes assessment tools facilitates the development of improved treatments for sarcoma patients. Results from major centers reveal that most patients with a nonmetastatic bone or soft tissue sarcoma will survive 5 years after surgery combined with either chemotherapy or radiation.

References

[1] Cheng EY, Springfield DS, Mankin HJ. Frequent incidence of extrapulmonary sites of initial metastasis in patients with liposarcoma. Cancer 1995;75(5):1120–7.

[2] Pearlstone DB, Pisters PW, Bold RJ, et al. Patterns of recurrence in extremity liposarcoma: implications for staging and follow-up. Cancer 1999;85(1):85–92.

[3] McMulkin HM, Yanchar NL, Fernandez CV, et al. Sentinel lymph node mapping and biopsy: a potentially valuable tool in the management of childhood extremity rhabdomyosarcoma. Pediatr Surg Int 2003;19(6):453–6.

[4] Blazer III DG, Sabel MS, Sondak VK. Is there a role for sentinel lymph node biopsy in the management of sarcoma? Surg Oncol 2003;12(3):201–6.

[5] Al-Refaie WB, Ali MW, Chu DZ, et al. Clear cell sarcoma in the era of sentinel lymph node mapping. J Surg Oncol 2004;87(3):126–9.

[6] Schuetze SM, Rubin BP, Vernon C, et al. Use of positron emission tomography in localized extremity soft tissue sarcoma treated with neoadjuvant chemotherapy. Cancer 2004;103(2): 339–48.
[7] Stroobants S, Goeminne J, Seegers M, et al. 18FDG-Positron emission tomography for the early prediction of response in advanced soft tissue sarcoma treated with imatinib mesylate (Glivec). Eur J Cancer 2003;39(14):2012–20.
[8] Kelloff GJ, Hoffman JM, Johnson B, et al. Progress and promise of FDG-PET imaging for cancer patient management and oncologic drug development. Clin Cancer Res 2005;11(8): 2785–808.
[9] Kelloff GJ, Bast Jr RC, Coffey DS, et al. Biomarkers, surrogate end points, and the acceleration of drug development for cancer prevention and treatment: an update prologue. Clin Cancer Res 2004;10(11):3881–4.
[10] Mankin HJ, Mankin CJ, Simon MA. The hazards of the biopsy, revisited. Members of the Musculoskeletal Tumor Society. J Bone Joint Surg Am 1996;78(5):656–63.
[11] Randall RL, Bruckner JD, Papenhausen MD, et al. Errors in diagnosis and margin determination of soft-tissue sarcomas initially treated at non-tertiary centers. Orthopedics 2004;27(2): 209–12.
[12] Gustafson P, Dreinhofer KE, Rydholm A. Soft tissue sarcoma should be treated at a tumor center. A comparison of quality of surgery in 375 patients. Acta Orthop Scand 1994;65(1):47–50.
[13] Munk PL, Vellet AD, Bramwell V, et al. Soft tissue sarcomas: a plea for proper management. Can J Surg 1993;36(2):178–80.
[14] Ozerdemoglu RA, Thompson Jr RC, Transfeldt EE, et al. Diagnostic value of open and needle biopsies in tumors of the sacrum. Spine 2003;28(9):909–15.
[15] Rodl RW, Hoffmann C, Gosheger G, et al. Ewing's sarcoma of the pelvis: combined surgery and radiotherapy treatment. J Surg Oncol 2003;83(3):154–60.
[16] Donaldson SS. Ewing sarcoma: radiation dose and target volume. Pediatr Blood Cancer 2004; 42(5):471–6.
[17] Dunst J, Schuck A. Role of radiotherapy in Ewing tumors. Pediatr Blood Cancer 2004; 42(5):465–70.
[18] Goorin AM, Schwartzentruber DJ, Devidas M, et al. Presurgical chemotherapy compared with immediate surgery and adjuvant chemotherapy for nonmetastatic osteosarcoma: Pediatric Oncology Group Study POG-8651. J Clin Oncol 2003;21(8):1574–80.
[19] Bacci G, Ferrari S, Longhi A, et al. Preoperative therapy versus immediate surgery in nonmetastatic osteosarcoma. J Clin Oncol 2003;21(24):4662–3.
[20] Cheng EY, Dusenbery KE, Winters MR, et al. Soft tissue sarcomas: preoperative versus postoperative radiation therapy. J Surg Oncol 1996;61:90–9.
[21] Eilber FC, Eilber FR, Eckardt J, et al. The impact of chemotherapy on the survival of patients with high-grade primary extremity liposarcoma. Ann Surg 2004;240(4):686–95 [discussion 695–7].
[22] Pisters PW, Harrison LB, Leung DH, et al. Long-term results of a prospective randomized trial of adjuvant brachytherapy in soft tissue sarcoma. J Clin Oncol 1996;14(3):859–68.
[23] Patel SR, Vadhan-Raj S, Burgess MA, et al. Preoperative chemotherapy with dose-intensive adriamycin (A) and ifosfamide (I) for high-risk primary soft-tissue sarcomas (STS) of extremity origin. Presented at the Connective Tissue Oncology Society. Arlington (VA), October 21–23, 1999.
[24] Bertoldo U, Brach del Prever EM, Gino G, et al. The integration of vascular surgical techniques with oncological surgical protocols in the treatment of soft tissue sarcomas of the limbs. Chir Organi Mov 2003;88(2):217–23.
[25] Bonardelli S, Nodari F, Maffeis R, et al. Limb salvage in lower-extremity sarcomas and technical details about vascular reconstruction. J Orthop Sci 2000;5(6):555–60.
[26] Hohenberger P, Allenberg JR, Schlag PM, et al. Results of surgery and multimodal therapy for patients with soft tissue sarcoma invading to vascular structures. Cancer 1999;85(2): 396–408.
[27] Zagars GK, Ballo MT, Pisters PW, et al. Surgical margins and reresection in the management

of patients with soft tissue sarcoma using conservative surgery and radiation therapy. Cancer 2003;97(10):2544–53.
[28] Davis AM, Kandel RA, Wunder JS, et al. The impact of residual disease on local recurrence in patients treated by initial unplanned resection for soft tissue sarcoma of the extremity. J Surg Oncol 1997;66(2):81–7.
[29] Cheng EY, Clohisy DR, Thompson RC. Soft tissue sarcomas: management of the patient after prior excisional biopsy. Presented at the Combined Meeting of the North American and European Musculoskeletal Tumor Societies. Boston, October 28–31, 1992.
[30] Noria S, Davis A, Kandel R, et al. Residual disease following unplanned excision of soft-tissue sarcoma of an extremity. J Bone Joint Surg Am 1996;78-A(5):650–5.
[31] Enneking WF, Spanier SS, Goodman MA. A system for the surgical staging of musculoskeletal sarcoma. Clin Orthop 1980;153:106–20.
[32] McKee MD, Liu DF, Brooks JJ, et al. The prognostic significance of margin width for extremity and trunk sarcoma. J Surg Oncol 2004;85(2):68–76.
[33] O'Sullivan B, Davis AM, Turcotte R, et al. Preoperative versus postoperative radiotherapy in soft-tissue sarcoma of the limbs: a randomised trial. Lancet 2002;359(9325):2235–41.
[34] Hsu HC, Huang EY, Wang CJ. Treatment results and prognostic factors in patients with malignant fibrous histiocytoma. Acta Oncol 2004;43(6):530–5.
[35] Frustaci S, De Paoli A, Bidoli E, et al. Ifosfamide in the adjuvant therapy of soft tissue sarcomas. Oncology 2003;65(Suppl 2):80–4.
[36] Stojadinovic A, Leung DH, Allen P, et al. Primary adult soft tissue sarcoma: time-dependent influence of prognostic variables. J Clin Oncol 2002;20(21):4344–52.
[37] Stefanovski PD, Bidoli E, De Paoli A, et al. Prognostic factors in soft tissue sarcomas: a study of 395 patients. Eur J Surg Oncol 2002;28(2):153–64.
[38] Trovik CS, Bauer HC, Berlin O, et al. Local recurrence of deep-seated, high-grade, soft tissue sarcoma: 459 patients from the Scandinavian Sarcoma Group Register. Acta Orthop Scand 2001;72(2):160–6.
[39] Stojadinovic A, Leung DH, Hoos A, et al. Analysis of the prognostic significance of microscopic margins in 2,084 localized primary adult soft tissue sarcomas. Ann Surg 2002;235(3):424–34.
[40] Pisters PW, Leung DH, Woodruff J, et al. Analysis of prognostic factors in 1,041 patients with localized soft tissue sarcomas of the extremities. J Clin Oncol 1996;14(5):1679–89.
[41] Trovik CS, Gustafson P, Bauer HC, et al. Consequences of local recurrence of soft tissue sarcoma: 205 patients from the Scandinavian Sarcoma Group Register. Acta Orthop Scand 2000;71(5):488–95.
[42] Kattan MW, Heller G, Brennan MF. A competing-risks nomogram for sarcoma-specific death following local recurrence. Stat Med 2003;22(22):3515–25.
[43] Eilber FC, Brennan MF, Eilber FR, et al. Validation of the postoperative nomogram for 12-year sarcoma-specific mortality. Cancer 2004;101(10):2270–5.
[44] Mariani L, Miceli R, Kattan MW, et al. Validation and adaptation of a nomogram for predicting the survival of patients with extremity soft tissue sarcoma using a three-grade system. Cancer 2005;103(2):402–8.
[45] Kattan MW, Leung DH, Brennan MF. Postoperative nomogram for 12-year sarcoma-specific death. J Clin Oncol 2002;20(3):791–6.
[46] Enneking W. Modification of the system for functional evaluation in the surgical management of musculoskeletal tumors. In: Enneking W, editor. Limb salvage in musculoskeletal oncology. New York: Churchill Livingston; 1987. p. 626–39.
[47] Davis AM, Wright JG, Williams JI, et al. Development of a measure of physical function for patients with bone and soft tissue sarcoma. Qual Life Res 1996;5(5):508–16.
[48] Getty PJ, Peabody TD. Complications and functional outcomes of reconstruction with an osteoarticular allograft after intra-articular resection of the proximal aspect of the humerus. J Bone Joint Surg Am 1999;81(8):1138–46.
[49] Kumar D, Grimer RJ, Abudu A, et al. Endoprosthetic replacement of the proximal humerus. Long-term results. J Bone Joint Surg Br 2003;85(5):717–22.

[50] Wittig JC, Bickels J, Kellar-Graney KL, et al. Osteosarcoma of the proximal humerus: long-term results with limb-sparing surgery. Clin Orthop Relat Res 2002;(397):156–76.

[51] Malo M, Davis AM, Wunder J, et al. Functional evaluation in distal femoral endoprosthetic replacement for bone sarcoma. Clin Orthop Relat Res 2001;(389):173–80.

[52] Schindler OS, Cannon SR, Briggs TW, et al. Stanmore custom-made extendible distal femoral replacements. Clinical experience in children with primary malignant bone tumours. J Bone Joint Surg Br 1997;79(6):927–37.

[53] Mankin HJ. The changes in major limb reconstruction as a result of the development of allografts. Chir Organi Mov 2003;88(2):101–13.

[54] Bickels J, Wittig JC, Kollender Y, et al. Distal femur resection with endoprosthetic reconstruction: a long-term followup study. Clin Orthop Relat Res 2002;(400):225–35.

[55] Davis AM, O'Sullivan B, Bell RS, et al. Function and health status outcomes in a randomized trial comparing preoperative and postoperative radiotherapy in extremity soft tissue sarcoma. J Clin Oncol 2002;20(22):4472–7.

[56] Bickels J, Wittig JC, Kollender Y, et al. Sciatic nerve resection: is that truly an indication for amputation? Clin Orthop Relat Res 2002;(399):201–4.

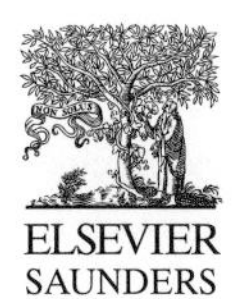

ELSEVIER
SAUNDERS

Hematol Oncol Clin N Am
19 (2005) 471–487

HEMATOLOGY/
ONCOLOGY
CLINICS OF
NORTH AMERICA

Imaging and Response in Soft Tissue Sarcomas

Scott M. Schuetze, MD, PhD

Division of Hematology/Oncology, Box 0848, University of Michigan Comprehensive Cancer Center, 1500 East Medical Center Drive, Ann Arbor, MI 48109-0848, USA

The objective radiographic response of tumor to chemotherapy is often used as a surrogate measure of therapeutic benefit to more rapidly evaluate the effectiveness of the treatment under investigation. Response, defined as a decrease in the size of the lesions, is thought to correlate with a decrease in the number of viable malignant cells and indicate the antitumor biologic activities of drugs or radiation. Enlargement of a tumor mass during therapy indicates growth of tumor that is resistant to drug or ionizing radiation. Recently, the convention for determining tumor response to treatment that was adopted by the World Health Organization (WHO) in 1981 was superseded by the guidelines established by the international Response Evaluation Criteria in Solid Tumors (RECIST) Group [1]. Most current trials of anticancer drugs that are given to patients who have advanced disease track changes in the sum of the longest dimension of target lesions to ascertain the rate of objective tumor response to treatment. RECIST provides a simple means for comparing tumor response results from different institutions, countries, and trials.

Sarcomas are a heterogenous group of malignant neoplasms that are derived from connective tissues. More than 50 types are recognized in the WHO classification of soft tissue tumors. Certain types of sarcomas, such as monophasic synovial sarcoma, are composed principally of malignant cells, whereas other types, such as myxofibrosarcoma, exhibit varying degrees of cellularity, fibrous septa, myxoid stroma, and necrosis. Intratumoral hemorrhage, inflammatory infiltrate, and cystic degeneration can also contribute to the size of sarcomas. Even if the neoplastic cells are effectively eradicated by therapy, the size of the heterogeneous tumor mass may not shrink or may enlarge as a result of induced necrosis or hemorrhage [2]. Therefore, RECIST may not accurately

E-mail address: scotschu@med.umich.edu

doi:10.1016/j.hoc.2005.03.001 ***hemonc.theclinics.com***

reflect the number of viable malignant cells present within the tumor mass. Changes in the tissue composition of a sarcoma, which can be assessed by histology or newer imaging modalities, may better reflect the biologic status of the malignancy, and therefore the effectiveness of the intervention, than do changes in tumor size [3]. In addition, treatment with active agents that target specific cellular signals may only suppress tumor growth rather than result in apoptosis and an objective response. In soft tissue sarcomas, measures of tumor response other than a change in size are likely to be more accurate predictors of a survival benefit from treatment.

The extent of disease within a patient and the likelihood of obtaining long-term remission after treatment currently influence clinicians' recommendations for systemic therapy. For example, many patients who have localized, high-grade soft tissue sarcomas of the extremity are at significant risk for disease recurrence because of hematogenous spread of tumor and are not cured by resection of disease. The risk for developing metastases rises with increasing size of the primary tumor such that high-grade soft tissue sarcomas more than 5 cm in greatest dimension have a more than 30% risk for recurrence within 5 years of surgery [4]. Because of the high likelihood of developing metastasis, many of the contemporary treatment protocols for stage III soft tissue sarcomas use multiple cycles of toxic doses of an anthracycline and ifosfamide even though few patients will benefit from treatment. Recently, chemotherapy protocols have been applied to the neoadjuvant treatment of localized soft tissue sarcomas in an effort to identify the patients who are likely to derive benefit from systemic therapy. Many of these studies have analyzed the association of radiographic changes with histopathologic findings, but only a few have investigated the correlation of radiographic or histologic changes with the risk for soft tissue sarcoma recurrence or death from disease [3,5].

In the setting of incurable advanced disease, the prolonged use of well-tolerated agents to suppress tumor growth and spread may be more desirable than the use of toxic chemotherapy to induce an objective response. Time to progression of disease or progression-free survival may be more important endpoints than tumor response in phase 2 studies of new agents for treatment of advanced sarcoma [6]. However, tumor progression by RECIST is defined in part by change in tumor size [1]. Studies correlating radiographic changes of localized or widespread sarcomas induced by chemotherapy or radiotherapy with survival outcomes are emerging and are the topic of this review. The following discussion does not address the use of histopathologic or molecular changes as potential surrogate measures of clinical benefit.

Conventional CT and MRI

CT and MRI are commonly used to evaluate changes in tumor size during chemotherapy. However, the response of soft tissue sarcomas has not consistently correlated with patient outcomes, and the optimal definition of response is not known. Multiple randomized trials comparing chemotherapy regimens for the treatment of advanced soft tissue sarcomas have shown significant differences in response rates but no difference in survival [7,8]. Possible explanations for the discrepancy between tumor response and survival outcomes include differences in patient care after documentation of disease progression or termination of the treatment phase of the study; differences in the rate of fatal toxicities; and the inability of conventional tumor imaging modalities to accurately depict changes in the biologic activity of sarcomas in response to systemic treatment.

Studies of the biologic effects of therapy on sarcomas are often more easily done when treatment is given pre-operatively and a sufficient amount of tissue is available for histologic and molecular analysis. The relationship between changes in the size or tissue viability of sarcomas and patient outcomes has been repeatedly evaluated in trials of neoadjuvant/adjuvant chemotherapy given to patients who have localized, resectable disease. One of the early studies found a significant correlation between tumor response and improved distant recurrence-free and overall survival [9]. This retrospective study abstracted information from records of approximately 46 patients who had localized, high-grade soft tissue sarcomas and were treated before 1986 with multiple cycles of cyclophosphamide, doxorubicin, and dacarbazine with or without vincristine before surgery. Response was defined as a 15% or more reduction in the cross-sectional area of the tumor derived from the greatest two-dimensional measurements recorded. Details of the imaging techniques used to determine tumor size were not described but included CT, ultrasound, and clinical measurement. CT was used in most cases. After a median follow-up of nearly 5 years, 64% of patients who had a tumor response were alive in contrast to 37% of patients who did not have a response to chemotherapy. A significant limitation of the study was that more than 50% of the patients presenting to the institution did not receive pre-operative chemotherapy because of physician bias, and therefore were not included in the analysis. The selection bias to not offer chemotherapy to some of the patients may have significantly influenced the study results. In addition, patients were not subjected to similar imaging studies or treated in a uniform manner. Many of the patients who were believed to not have a response to pre-operative treatment had early termination of systemic therapy and did not receive adjuvant chemotherapy, whereas most of the patients who were thought to have responding tumors received multiple cycles of adjuvant in addition to neoadjuvant chemotherapy. A subsequent retrospective analysis of a subset of patients who had localized primary or recurrent high-grade or large (≥ 5 cm in size) soft tissue sarcomas, were mostly treated with a doxorubicin-containing regimen after 1990, and underwent imaging of the tumor using contemporary CT or MRI scanners, identified a correlation between a radiographic response to neoadjuvant chemotherapy and overall survival [10]. However, tumor response did not correlate with local recurrence-free survival in multivariate analysis and the effect (or lack thereof) of tumor response on distance recurrence of sarcoma was not mentioned. The improvement in survival in the group of patients who had a response could have been caused by factors unrelated to sarcoma. The investigators calculated tumor volume by multiplying the craniocaudal, anteroposterior, and transverse dimensions and scored a decrease in tumor volume of 15% or more as a response to chemotherapy. Major shortcomings of the study are that more than five different chemotherapy regimens were used neoadjuvantly, the use of adjuvant chemotherapy was not discussed, and survival follow-up was a short median of 3 years. Prospective studies of four cycles of neoadjuvant etoposide, ifosfamide, and doxorubicin combined with regional hyperthermia have been performed on patients who have high-risk retroperitoneal, visceral, or extremity soft tissue sarcomas to determine the response rate of this combined modality treatment and its effect on patient survival [11,12]. Response was defined unusually as a decrease in the cross-sectional area of tumor of 25% or more or 75% or more necrosis within the primary tumor mass assessed by standard pathology at the time of surgery. Patients who had tumor response to pre-operative therapy had a significantly lower risk for death with a median follow-up of nearly 7 years, but the investigators did not discuss whether tumor response correlated with a lower risk for local recurrence in patients who had completely resected disease or a lower risk for developing metastasis. Moreover, the investigators did not report whether there was a significant correlation between tumor response, determined by radiographic means alone, and patient survival.

The definition of tumor response in the above studies was broad. The definitions of response established by the RECIST group and used in many of the current trials of chemotherapy in advanced disease are substantially more restrictive. For example, an objective response by RECIST corresponds to a decrease of more than 50% in the cross-sectional area and more than 65% in the volume of tumor [13]. An apparent change in tumor volume of 10% to 20% is within the range of interobserver variability and may not reflect a true change in the size of a lesion [14]. The optimal radiographic criteria with which to differentiate responsive versus resistant disease are not known. The number of well-planned, prospective studies correlating changes in tumor size or volume during chemotherapy with unequivocal progression of disease, risk for disease recurrence, and patient survival are limited.

Several studies have refuted claims of an association between sarcoma response and survival. A comprehensive retrospective review of a large number (N = 76) of patients presenting with stage III soft tissue sarcoma of the extremity who were treated with neoadjuvant chemotherapy failed to find a significant correlation between response and distant metastasis-free, disease-free, or overall survival [15]. The type of scan used to assess response was not discussed but was presumably an MRI in most cases. A lack of correlation between tumor response and improved patient outcomes was observed whether patients who had a minor response to therapy were scored as nonresponders in keeping with RECIST, or as responders as in the prior analysis by Pezzi et al [9]. The authors concluded that the decision to prescribe adjuvant treatment should not be based on tumor response to pre-operative chemotherapy assessed by conventional radiographic imaging. Other studies of neoadjuvant treatment of localized sarcomas have also failed to identify a significant correlation between tumor response and patient outcome [5,16]. In the trial conducted by Delaney et al [5], 48 patients who had extremity, high-grade soft tissue sarcomas that were 8 cm or more in size were prospectively treated pre-operatively with three cycles of doxorubicin, ifosfamide, and dacarbazine interdigitated with a total of 44 Gy of radiotherapy. Using RECIST, the authors classified 10.6%, 76.6%, and 12.8% of patients as having a partial response, stable disease, and progression of disease, respectively. Response was determined by comparing tumor size on an MRI obtained at the completion of pre-operative chemoradiotherapy with tumor size on a baseline MRI obtained at study entry before initiation of treatment. Radiologic response did not correlate with metastasis-free, disease-free, or overall survival. Moreover, in four of the six patients who had progression of disease, the excised tumor was 90% or more necrotic, suggesting tumor was biologically sensitive to the cytotoxic effects of chemotherapy or radiation.

Because many sarcomas contain a heterogeneous composition of malignant cells, supporting stroma, and necrotic or hemorrhagic tissue contained within a pseudocapsule, complete responses are seldom seen and the size of the tumor mass frequently does not reflect the degree of viable malignancy. Necrotic, hemorrhagic, or cystic regions within a tumor can be distinguished from more solid, cellular areas containing viable neoplasia using CT or MRI. However, it seems the relationship between changes in the absolute or relative density of tissue within a sarcoma mass and risk for recurrence of disease or death has not been published. Newer imaging modalities may be better able than standard CT or MRI to differentiate regions of viable from nonviable tumor and may prove to be useful for detecting clinically meaningful tumor response to treatment.

Positron emission tomography

Positron emission tomography (PET) is able to use various radiopharmaceuticals to visualize and quantify different biologic properties of tumors in vivo. The radioactive tracers used in PET generate positrons that collide with nearby electrons. The interaction annihilates the particles generating two 511 keV gamma-rays that travel in 180° opposite directions. PET scanners are able to register the simultaneously produced gamma-rays traveling within the field of view of the detector and provide spatial representation of the distribution of tracer. Image quality and resolution are better when dedicated PET scanners are used, and correction for attenuation of gamma-rays through tissue of varying thickness and composition using an external radiation source is necessary to derive reproducible, semiquantitative, and quantitative results. The maximum and average pixel density within a specified region of interest can be determined and adjusted by the quantity of tracer administered and body weight to calculate the maximum standardized uptake value (SUV) and average SUV, respectively. The degree of heterogeneity of radiotracer distribution within a tumor can also be quantified and may provide additional information about the biology of tumors [17]. Several different radioactive tracers including 18F-fluorodeoxyglucose (FDG) [18–20], 18F-fluoromisonidazole [21], 18F-fluorodeoxythymidine [22], 11C-thymidine [23], 11C-tyrosine [24], and11C-choline [25] to measure glycolysis, hypoxia, DNA synthesis, DNA synthesis, protein synthesis, and biosynthesis of cell membranes, respectively, have been studied in humans who have soft tissue sarcomas using PET, but the bulk of available data is from the use of FDG.

FDG is a glucose analog that is actively transported into cells, is phosphorylated, and does not undergo further metabolism in the glycolytic pathway, thus remaining an intracellularly trapped, radioactive tracer. High-grade soft tissue sarcomas accumulate FDG more than resting muscle, normal connective tissue, and many organs, presumably because of increased requirements for energy. In sarcomas, the degree of FDG uptake correlates with tumor cellularity and proliferation [26]. Eary et al [27] first studied sarcomas using FDG PET, relating the quantitative value of the FDG metabolic rate of tumor (MRFDG) to the semiquantitative measure of tumor uptake, the SUV. The MRFDG was determined by precise dynamic imaging with serial blood sampling and graphical data analysis. This validation of the tumor SUV in sarcomas set the stage for determining sarcoma treatment response using SUV. The tumor maximum SUV correlates positively with tumor grade and is likely to be a more useful value than the average SUV in higher grade sarcomas because the maximum value is not diminished by the presence of large areas of necrosis or hemorrhage [28]. Changes in FDG accumulation within a sarcoma may be a useful measure of changes in tumor activity and viability.

High levels of circulating insulin can enhance FDG uptake in normal tissues, and hyperglycemia can decrease FDG uptake in a sarcoma because of competition from glucose for transport into tumor cells. Therefore, FDG PET imaging should be performed after at least 6 hours of fasting, and a prescan blood glucose level should be obtained if SUV measurements are to be compared between sequential studies in the same patient or between patients. The European Organization for Research and Treatment of Cancer (EORTC) generated consensus guidelines in 1999 for the measurement of tumor response using FDG and PET in an effort to standardize basic techniques involved in PET imaging to allow for comparisons across studies [29]. The objective was to provide a framework for neoadjuvant studies so that comparable FDG PET methods were applied to response assessments. However, most of the available data regarding changes in FDG uptake in sarcomas has been collected before publication of the guidelines.

Near simultaneous reports exploring the potential correlation of changes in FDG uptake in sarcomas of soft tissue treated with isolated limb perfusion (ILP) or radiation were published in 1996 [19,20]. Van Ginkel et al [20] studied 20 patients who had locally advanced sarcomas of the extremity. The investigators performed FDG PET scans before, 2 weeks after, and 8 weeks after ILP, and compared the PET results with histologic findings after careful examination of macroscopic and microscopic changes in tumor. Patients had fasted for at least 6 hours and blood glucose levels were normal at the time of PET scanning. Images were corrected for signal attenuation. The rate of FDG uptake was determined for the most active portion, the rim, and the core of the tumor. Seven patients had a complete pathologic response, 12 patients had a partial pathologic response, and tumor was not excised in one patient because of rapid progression of disease in distant sites. FDG uptake in tumor declined more than 75% from baseline within 2 weeks after ILP in five of the seven patients and within 8 weeks after ILP in six of the seven patients who had a complete histologic response. The largest decrements in FDG uptake occurred within 2 weeks after ILP, and additional declines in glucose uptake between weeks 2 and 8 were minor. Even though the patients who had complete responses had dramatic declines in glucose uptake within the tumor mass, the rate of FDG accumulation remained above background levels in the pseudocapsules because of infiltration of inflammatory cells. In one patient who had a complete pathologic response of a low-grade myxoid liposarcoma, there was little change in a low rate of FDG accumulation after ILP. FDG uptake increased in one patient, declined less than 50% in six patients, and declined less than 75% but more than 50% in four patients who had partial pathologic responses. In seven of the patients who had partial pathologic responses, viable tumor remained in the pseudocapsules and was detected by FDG PET. In the other patients who had partial responses, regions within the tumor mass remained FDG avid. FDG activity in the rim of tumor with a partial pathologic response was caused by the presence of an inflammatory infiltrate and viable tumor coexisting in the vascular pseudocapsule. The investigators concluded that significant declines in sarcoma glucose metabolism occur within 2 weeks of ILP but that FDG PET cannot distinguish a complete from a partial response based on the absolute rate of FDG uptake. The investigators did not address whether the relative degree of decline in glucose metabolism, rather than the absolute value, may be more predictive of a complete pathologic response. Substitution of L-1-11C-tyrosine for FDG to monitor changes in protein synthesis in sarcomas treated with ILP using PET has discriminated between residual viable tumor and inflammation within a pseudocapsule and may be a better radiotracer than FDG to monitor sarcoma response to ILP. However, experience with this agent in sarcomas is limited [24].

Jones et al [19] studied changes in FDG uptake in a small set of four patients treated for soft tissue sarcoma using radiation and hyperthermia. Patients fasted 4 hours before the PET studies and blood glucose values were normal at the time of FDG injection. The investigators generated attenuation-corrected images and performed PET scans before and at the completion of therapy in three of the patients. Tumor maximum SUVs were calculated from the pretreatment scans and ranged from 2.6 to 12. Moderate enlargement in the central area of tumor showing absence of FDG uptake was seen in two of the patients and a minor change in FDG uptake was seen in one of the patients. Changes in the maximum SUV were not reported. Absent or diminished uptake on PET correlated with pathologic necrosis of tumor. The study was too small to draw conclusions about the correlation between changes in FDG uptake and tumor response. Neither Jones et al [19] or Ginkel et al [20] reported on disease recurrence.

Eary and coworkers [18] found that a higher tumor maximum SUV at diagnosis correlated with a greater risk for disease progression and death from disease in patients who had soft tissue or bone sarcomas. Moreover, by multivariate analysis and independent of tumor type, tumor grade, and patient age, the tumor maximum SUV predicted survival in a dose-dependent manner, suggesting that the tumor SUV is related to the biologic aggressiveness of sarcomas. A subsequent study of serial FDG PET in a homogeneous population of patients who had high-grade, extremity soft tissue sarcomas to investigate the correlation between changes in tumor SUV and outcomes was recently reported [30]. In this study, 46 patients were imaged before treatment and after two, three, or four cycles of doxorubicin-based, multiagent chemotherapy and were followed for disease recurrence and survival. Patients fasted for at least 6 hours and blood glucose levels were less than 120 mg/dL before PET scanning. The correlation of objective radiographic response using conventional MRI or CT and outcomes was not analyzed. Patients who had a pretreatment tumor maximum SUV that was six or more had a significantly higher risk for disease recurrence than patients who had less FDG avid sarcomas. An FDG PET response was defined as a reduction of the maximum tumor SUV of 40% or more from the pretreatment value. Patients who had evidence of an FDG PET response to neoadjuvant chemotherapy had a significantly lower risk for disease recurrence and death from disease. On multivariate analysis, the pretreatment tumor maximum SUV and the change in maximum SUV after neoadjuvant chemotherapy correlated independently with disease-free and metastasis-free survival. A 75% disease-free survival and 80% overall survival rate at 5 years from diagnosis was estimated for the 12 patients who had a baseline maximum SUV of six or more and an FDG PET response to chemotherapy. In comparison, patients who had a baseline maximum SUV of six or more and no FDG PET response had an estimated 5-year disease-free survival of 15% and overall survival of 35%. FDG PET may be able to discriminate the patients who have high-grade soft tissue sarcomas and are more likely to derive benefit from chemotherapy from the patients in whom the long-term prognosis is poor. The findings need to be confirmed by a larger, multi-institutional study before FDG PET should be used routinely to guide chemotherapeutic decisions.

Dynamic contrast-enhanced MRI

Dynamic contrast-enhanced MRI (DCE-MRI) uses bolus administration of a water soluble and paramagnetic contrast, rapidly obtained magnetic resonance sequences, and complex software to measure tissue characteristics related to vascular perfusion and diffusion. A principal advantage of DCE-MRI is that the method can distinguish regions of viable tumor from reparative changes and nonvital tissue. During the first pass of a small molecule contrast agent through the capillaries of tumor, rapid diffusion of the agent into the interstitial compartment occurs because of increased vessel density, high perfusion rates, and increased capillary permeability [31]. Viable tumor enhances rapidly following intravenous injection of contrast, whereas areas of necrosis, cystic degeneration, hemorrhage, and fibrosis enhance more slowly. The differences in the rate of enhancement between regions of tumor containing viable neoplasia and devitalized tissues can be measured by obtaining serial MRI sequences beginning within seconds after rate-controlled bolus administration of contrast. The technique yields semiquantitative data, but results may become quantitative as the models of perfusion/diffusion kinetics improve. The rapidity with which the sequences must be acquired to determine the kinetics of contrast diffusion often required that a specific region of interest be identified before administration of contrast. Dynamic analysis of contrast enhancement has usually been limited to one imaging plane that was predetermined by the radiologist after selecting a region of interest within the tumor mass using conventional MRI techniques. Recent advances in technology allow for a larger volume of tumor to be imaged during dynamic contrast-enhancement, which may minimize potential bias introduced by the radiologist. However, a large volume of tumor encompassed by MRI scans usually sacrifices spatial resolution in the images. DCE-MRI measures changes in certain aspects of tumor physiology, such as capillary density and permeability. These changes are likely to precede changes in tumor volume and may serve as an early indication of response to treatment but can also be nonspecific. DCE-MRI to assess response to chemotherapy was initially performed in osteosarcoma and Ewing's sarcoma, but is beginning to be applied to the study of soft tissue sarcomas [32–34].

Soft tissue sarcoma response to treatment characterized by DCE-MRI has been correlated to histologic findings, but it seems the relationship between changes in early enhancement of tumor and risk for recurrence or death from disease has not been reported [35–38]. Shapeero et al [36] briefly described their experience with DCE-MRI in 32 patients who had soft tissue sarcoma and underwent imaging before and after neoadjuvant chemotherapy. The persistence of regions of early contrast enhancement that nearly coincided temporally with enhancement of arteries after treatment correlated with the presence of more than 10% residual viable tumor. However, the investigators did not report whether the images were matched to histologic analysis to determine if early enhancement localized to the regions containing viable neoplasia posttreatment. The absence of early enhancing tissue correlated with a good histologic response (defined as less than 10% residual viable tumor) to therapy. Details of the histologic type, stage, and location of sarcomas that were treated and the chemotherapy regimen and statistical methods that were used were not reported. Because of the limited discussion of the patient population and results, it is difficult to determine whether DCE-MRI correlates with histologic response in a select population of patients who have soft tissue sarcoma or is potentially more widely applicable.

More recently, DCE-MRI has been studied in patients undergoing ILP for treatment of high-grade sarcomas of the extremities [37,38]. Van Rijswijk and collaborators [37] prospectively studied 12 patients referred for ILP with DCE-MRI to evaluate whether changes in the kinetics of tissue enhancement correlated with changes in the size of tumor or amount of viable tumor at surgery and whether areas of persistent rapid enhancement colocalized with residual viable neoplasia after treatment. The affected limb was perfused with tumor necrosis factor α and melphalan in all 12 of the patients. One patient did not undergo a second DCE-MRI because an amputation was performed 2 days after initiating ILP to manage necrosis of the hand, and one patient was not a candidate for definitive surgery because of the rapid development of pulmonary metastasis. In the other ten patients, the second DCE-MRI was performed a median of 2 months after ILP and surgery was performed a median of 1 month after the second MRI. Tumor was considered to contain viable neoplasia if rapid contrast enhancement occurred early after administration of gadolinium. A complete dynamic MRI response, partial dynamic MRI response, and no change in MRI response were defined as the absence of early rapid enhancement, early enhancement in less than 50% of the remnant mass, and early enhancement in 50% or more of the remnant mass, respectively. A partial clinical response was defined as a decrease in tumor volume of 35% or more, progressive disease was defined as an increase in tumor volume of more than 35%, and clinical response was scored as no change if the change in volume did not meet criteria for partial response or progressive disease. Histologic response was defined as complete if no residual viable tumor was present, partial if less than 50% of the tumor mass contained viable-appearing neoplasia, and no change if 50% or more of the remnant mass contained viable tumor. All of the patients had early contrast enhancement of regions within the tumor before ILP. The histologic findings met the criteria for partial response in five patients, and no change in five patients. All five of the patients who had no histologic change to ILP had no change by DCE-MRI, whereas three of the patients who had partial histologic response had a partial response in DCE-MRI, and the other two patients had complete disappearance of early contrast enhancement. A change in the size of tumor did not correlate with histologic response. The pattern of enhancement (multifocal versus peripheral) appeared to correlate with the location of residual viable tumor. Late, gradual, or absence of contrast enhancement was seen in areas containing necrosis, granulation tissue, or fibrosis.

Another prospective study of DCE-MRI to monitor response to ILP in 18 patients was reported by Vanel et al [38]. Sixteen of the patients underwent DCE-MRI before, 1 month after, and 2 months after ILP. DCE-MRI showing tissue enhancement that was temporally similar to arterial enhancement within the tumor mass was scored as viable tumor present. A lack of rapid enhancement of tissue was scored as absence of viable tumor. The investigators compared qualitative changes in tumor enhancement. After ILP, three patients had lack of active tumor by DCE-MRI, of which two had complete pathologic response and one had diffusely infiltrating, viable-appearing neoplasia but no discrete mass. Six patients had enlargement of a nonenhancing central area within the mass and persistence of enhancement seen as a thin rim surrounding the sarcoma. In five of the six patients, necrosis was present in more than 98% of the specimen at surgery. The study did not describe whether the enhancing thin rim contained viable tumor within a pseudocapsule. In three patients, after an initial improvement in tumor enhancement, an enhancing rim of tissue thickened into a wall between 1 and 2 months after ILP and active tumor within the wall was seen histologically. In four patients, enhancement of some of the nodules persisted after ILP and pathology confirmed the presence of viable tumor. With the exception of the three patients who had an initial good response followed by growth of tumor in the periphery of the mass, the investigators did not discuss the time-course of change in tumor enhancement measured by DCE-MRI after ILP, but this aspect should be investigated to determine whether patients would benefit from surgery performed earlier after ILP.

Because ILP is local-regional therapy, the dynamic MRI response to treatment is not likely to correlate with distant recurrence of disease or overall survival. The usefulness of DCE-MRI in patients undergoing ILP may be in determining which patients should undergo amputation versus a limb-sparing procedure for local control of disease. Before DCE-MRI can be used to help guide therapeutic decisions about chemotherapy, it is necessary to develop standardized approaches to obtain and analyze dynamically acquired images, determine which characteristics of tumor enhancement are informative, and validate the methods using patient outcomes rather than histologic response. Because of the ability of DCE-MRI to differentiate viable sarcoma from necrosis, fibrosis, and degenerating tissue, additional neoadjuvant trials incorporating DCE-MRI to study whether changes in tumor vascularity are prognostic of outcome may be informative.

Magnetic resonance spectroscopy

Phosphorous-31 magnetic resonance spectroscopy (MRS) is a noninvasive tool that measures levels of energy rich phosphates (eg, adenosine triphosphate, phosphocreatinine); membrane-bound phosphomonoester and phosphodiester; and inorganic phosphate, and allows estimation of intracellular pH. Phosphorous MRS has been studied extensively in murine sarcoma models and preliminarily in human sarcomas [39]. Although an elevated (alkaline) tumor pH pretherapy has correlated with a high degree of tumor necrosis after hyperthermia and radiation [40], it has not been established whether the correlation exists because alkaline tumors are more inherently necrotic or because alkaline tumors respond better to radiation. Several trials suggest that reduction in phosphomonoester or phosphodiester after treatment of sarcoma correlates with pathologic response or radiographic response [41–44]. However, it seems the association between changes in phosphate levels or pH and patient survival has not been reported. Further study of phosphorous MRS needs to be done before the technique can be integrated into sarcoma clinical management practices.

Thallium-201 scintigraphy

Thallium-201 chloride is a radionuclide potassium analog that is actively pumped into cells through the sodium-potassium adenosine triphosphate–dependent pump and is used routinely to image the heart. Thallium scintigraphy is a valuable tool to differentiate viable myocardium, which actively accumulates thallium chloride from infarcted myocardium or scar tissue that do not. Many soft tissue sarcomas uptake thallium at an increased rate compared with normal surrounding connective tissue. Qualitative changes in tumor uptake of thallium after treatment with chemotherapy or radiation therapy have correlated with histology [45,46]. Almost all of the residual sarcoma masses that had reduced uptake of thallium after treatment were composed of more than 90% necrotic tissue. All of the sarcomas with elevated accumulation of thallium after treatment had poor histologic responses. It seems an association between reduced thallium uptake and improved clinical outcomes has not yet been published. However, thallium scintigraphy may be useful to identify the sarcomas that are mostly unaffected by chemotherapy or radiotherapy, and presently is more widely available and less costly than PET.

Gastrointestinal stromal tumors

Chemotherapy for gastrointestinal stromal tumors (GIST) changed dramatically after the introduction of imatinib mesylate, a small molecule inhibitor of the abl, kit, and platelet-derived growth factor receptor tyrosine kinases, and is a paradigm for management of solid tumors using targeted systemic therapy. It has also been a model for study of the ability of functional imaging to predict molecular response and clinical outcomes in soft tissue sarcoma. Identification of activating mutations in the c-Kit receptor stimulating cell growth and inhibiting apoptosis promoted interest in the use of imatinib to block this aberrant signal in GIST. Trials of daily therapy with imatinib showed remarkably high activity with objective responses in more than 50% of patients [47,48]. The median time to objective response was 13 to 15 weeks. However, 10% to 15% of patients had progression of disease that was not evident by CT for up to 3 months after the start of imatinib. New agents are under development for the treatment of imatinib-resistant GIST. Therefore, a rapid means to predict resistance to imatinib will be desirable when additional effective targeted therapy becomes available.

The first report of imatinib activity in GIST described dramatic reduction in FDG uptake in lesions within 1 month of treatment [49]. Multiple groups have subsequently found that changes in FDG accumulation in GIST occur early after initiation of drug and often precede changes seen on CT [50–53]. Stroobants et al [53] described changes in symptoms attributed to tumor, tumor size, and FDG uptake in 19 patients who had GIST treated on a phase 1 or phase 2 trial of imatinib. The investigators performed FDG PET after a fast, attenuation-corrected the images, and followed the EORTC recommendations to assign response. The investigators performed the FDG PET before treatment, after 8 days, and after 28 days from the start of imatinib. Seventeen patients had elevated FDG uptake in GIST before treatment. Ten of the 17 patients had partial response by RECIST within 4 to 48 weeks. Thirteen of the patients had a complete or partial FDG PET response within 8 days. PET response preceded CT response by a median of 7 weeks. Progression of disease by PET (increase in the SUV of more than 25% in a target lesion or the appearance of new metabolically active tumors) was seen by day 8 in three patients, and no change in FDG accumulation was seen in one patient. RECIST progression of disease occurred in all four of the patients who did not have a PET response within 2 to 21 weeks (median 5 weeks) of starting drug therapy. Improvement in symptoms and FDG uptake in tumor correlated, and patients who had worsening FDG accumulation experienced clinical deterioration. Patients who had a FDG PET response of GIST to imatinib had a significantly longer time to progression by RECIST than patients who did not have a PET response. There is a confirmed concordance between improvement in FDG uptake 8 days after starting therapy and good clinical outcomes [52]. Moreover, there is a reported correlation between the absence of FDG uptake in GIST after starting therapy and improvement in survival [51]. FDG PET performed early after the start of imatinib is likely to be useful for identifying the patients who are at increased risk for progression of disease and should be considered for an alternative treatment. Studies to determine whether FDG PET more accurately predicts survival than CT are needed to support the principle that a metabolic change is more informative of the potential clinical benefit than a change in tumor size, at least in GIST.

Summary

The ability of RECIST to identify the sarcomas that are responding biologically to cytotoxic therapies is poor. Moreover, it has not been shown conclusively that RECIST response portends an improved clinical outcome, or conversely that lack of RECIST response is associated with earlier death from disease. Soft tissue sarcomas are a diverse group of neoplasms of which many are structurally complex. The heterogeneity of tissues that make up sarcomas and the highly vascular nature of high-grade lesions likely contribute significantly to the poor correlation of changes in tumor size with cellular responses to chemotherapy and radiotherapy.

Imaging modalities that measure biologic processes have been studied in sarcomas, but most of the studies have been exploratory in nature, the results are preliminary, and a correlation with clinical outcomes has not been reported with the exception of FDG PET. Nevertheless, functional imaging methods are promising means to depict important biologic changes in sarcomas in response to therapy. The treatment of extremity sarcomas using ILP has provided a platform of uniform treatment with which to study the ability of FDG PET, DCE-MRI, and MRS to predict pathologic response. A consistent finding was that a change in tumor size did not correlate with histologic response. A change in FDG uptake, the rate of tissue enhancement, and phosphomonoester levels correlated with histologic findings, thus functional imaging of a biologic process more accurately reflected tumor viability after ILP than conventional MRI. FDG PET may be the most useful of the three methods because of higher spatial resolution in the images, availability, and the ability to detect a response early after therapy. However, tumor necrosis factor is not widely available, and changes in the biologic parameters of sarcomas treated with ILP versus systemic chemotherapy may not be similar.

FDG PET findings have correlated with disease recurrence/progression and survival in extremity soft tissue sarcomas and GIST. These findings should be corroborated with larger multi-institutional trials and trials of other agents to determine whether PET is informative for a more diverse group of sarcoma patients. As more active drugs for the treatment of GIST become available clinically, PET may be the most useful method to monitor tumor response to therapy and influence therapeutic decisions. The ability of PET and other functional imaging modalities to detect early responses to therapy make them more suitable than RECIST to predict clinical outcomes from chemotherapy. A concerted effort to conduct appropriately designed clinical, multicenter studies is needed to replace tumor size with biochemical parameters in the assessment of response. The biochemical parameter and imaging modality most suited to measure response may be histology specific, thus identifiable only through cooperative efforts.

Acknowledgments

I thank Dr. Janet Eary for critically reviewing the manuscript and providing helpful suggestions.

References

[1] Therasse P, Arbuck SG, Eisenhauer EA, et al. New guidelines to evaluate the response to treatment in solid tumors. European Organization for Research and Treatment of Cancer, National Cancer Institute of the United States, National Cancer Institute of Canada. J Natl Cancer Inst 2000;92(3):205–16.

[2] Panicek DM, Casper ES, Brennan MF, et al. Hemorrhage simulating tumor growth in malignant fibrous histiocytoma at MR imaging. Radiology 1991;181(2):398–400.

[3] Eilber FC, Rosen G, Eckardt J, et al. Treatment-induced pathologic necrosis: a predictor of local recurrence and survival in patients receiving neoadjuvant therapy for high-grade extremity soft tissue sarcomas. J Clin Oncol 2001;19(13):3203–9.

[4] Pisters PW, Leung DH, Woodruff J, et al. Analysis of prognostic factors in 1,041 patients with localized soft tissue sarcomas of the extremities. J Clin Oncol 1996;14(5):1679–89.

[5] DeLaney TF, Spiro IJ, Suit HD, et al. Neoadjuvant chemotherapy and radiotherapy for large extremity soft-tissue sarcomas. Int J Radiat Oncol Biol Phys 2003;56(4):1117–27.

[6] Van Glabbeke M, Verweij J, Judson I, et al. Progression-free rate as the principal end-point for phase II trials in soft-tissue sarcomas. Eur J Cancer 2002;38(4):543–9.

[7] Antman K, Crowley J, Balcerzak SP, et al. An intergroup phase III randomized study of doxorubicin and dacarbazine with or without ifosfamide and mesna in advanced soft tissue and bone sarcomas. J Clin Oncol 1993;11(7):1276–85.

[8] Edmonson JH, Ryan LM, Blum RH, et al. Randomized comparison of doxorubicin alone versus ifosfamide plus doxorubicin or mitomycin, doxorubicin, and cisplatin against advanced soft tissue sarcomas. J Clin Oncol 1993;11(7):1269–75.

[9] Pezzi CM, Pollock RE, Evans HL, et al. Preoperative chemotherapy for soft-tissue sarcomas of the extremities. Ann Surg 1990;211(4):476–81.

[10] Meric F, Hess KR, Varma DG, et al. Radiographic response to neoadjuvant chemotherapy is a predictor of local control and survival in soft tissue sarcomas. Cancer 2002;95(5):1120–6.

[11] Issels RD, Abdel-Rahman S, Wendtner C, et al. Neoadjuvant chemotherapy combined with regional hyperthermia (RHT) for locally advanced primary or recurrent high-risk adult soft-tissue sarcomas (STS) of adults: long-term results of a phase II study. Eur J Cancer 2001; 37(13):1599–608.

[12] Wendtner CM, Abdel-Rahman S, Krych M, et al. Response to neoadjuvant chemotherapy combined with regional hyperthermia predicts long-term survival for adult patients with retroperitoneal and visceral high-risk soft tissue sarcomas. J Clin Oncol 2002;20(14):3156–64.

[13] James K, Eisenhauer E, Christian M, et al. Measuring response in solid tumors: unidimensional versus bidimensional measurement. J Natl Cancer Inst 1999;91(6):523–8.

[14] Schwartz LH, Ginsberg MS, DeCorato D, et al. Evaluation of tumor measurements in oncology: use of film-based and electronic techniques. J Clin Oncol 2000;18(10):2179–84.

[15] Pisters PW, Patel SR, Varma DG, et al. Preoperative chemotherapy for stage IIIB extremity soft tissue sarcoma: long-term results from a single institution. J Clin Oncol 1997;15(12): 3481–7.

[16] Casper ES, Gaynor JJ, Harrison LB, et al. Preoperative and postoperative adjuvant combination chemotherapy for adults with high grade soft tissue sarcoma. Cancer 1994;73(6):1644–51.

[17] O'Sullivan F, Roy S, Eary J. A statistical measure of tissue heterogeneity with application to 3D PET sarcoma data. Biostatistics 2003;4(3):433–48.

[18] Eary JF, O'Sullivan F, Powitan Y, et al. Sarcoma tumor FDG uptake measured by PET and patient outcome: a retrospective analysis. Eur J Nucl Med Mol Imaging 2002;29(9):1149–54.

[19] Jones DN, McCowage GB, Sostman HD, et al. Monitoring of neoadjuvant therapy response of soft-tissue and musculoskeletal sarcoma using fluorine-18-FDG PET. J Nucl Med 1996; 37(9):1438–44.

[20] van Ginkel RJ, Hoekstra HJ, Pruim J, et al. FDG-PET to evaluate response to hyperthermic isolated limb perfusion for locally advanced soft-tissue sarcoma. J Nucl Med 1996;37(6): 984–90.

[21] Rajendran JG, Wilson DC, Conrad EU, et al. [(18)F]FMISO and [(18)F]FDG PET imaging in soft tissue sarcomas: correlation of hypoxia, metabolism and VEGF expression. Eur J Nucl Med Mol Imaging 2003;30(5):695–704.

[22] Cobben DC, Elsinga PH, Suurmeijer AJ, et al. Detection and grading of soft tissue sarcomas of the extremities with (18)F-3′-fluoro-3′-deoxy-L-thymidine. Clin Cancer Res 2004;10(5): 1685–90.

[23] Shields AF, Mankoff DA, Link JM, et al. Carbon-11-thymidine and FDG to measure therapy response. J Nucl Med 1998;39(10):1757–62.

[24] van Ginkel RJ, Kole AC, Nieweg OE, et al. L-[1–11C]-tyrosine PET to evaluate response to hyperthermic isolated limb perfusion for locally advanced soft-tissue sarcoma and skin cancer. J Nucl Med 1999;40(2):262–7.

[25] Zhang H, Tian M, Oriuchi N, et al. 11C-choline PET for the detection of bone and soft tissue tumours in comparison with FDG PET. Nucl Med Commun 2003;24(3):273–9.

[26] Folpe AL, Lyles RH, Sprouse JT, et al. (F-18) fluorodeoxyglucose positron emission tomography as a predictor of pathologic grade and other prognostic variables in bone and soft tissue sarcoma. Clin Cancer Res 2000;6(4):1279–87.

[27] Eary JF, Mankoff DA. Tumor metabolic rates in sarcoma using FDG PET. J Nucl Med 1998;39(2):250–4.

[28] Eary JF, Conrad EU. Positron emission tomography in grading soft tissue sarcomas. Semin Musculoskelet Radiol 1999;3(2):135–8.

[29] Young H, Baum R, Cremerius U, et al. Measurement of clinical and subclinical tumour response using [18F]-fluorodeoxyglucose and positron emission tomography: review and 1999 EORTC recommendations. European Organization for Research and Treatment of Cancer (EORTC) PET Study Group. Eur J Cancer 1999;35(13):1773–82.

[30] Schuetze SM, Rubin BP, Vernon C, et al. Use of positron emission tomography in localized extremity soft tissue sarcoma treated with neoadjuvant chemotherapy. Cancer 2005;103(2): 339–48.

[31] Padhani AR, Husband JE. Dynamic contrast-enhanced MRI studies in oncology with an emphasis on quantification, validation and human studies. Clin Radiol 2001;56(8):607–20.

[32] Brisse H, Ollivier L, Edeline V, et al. Imaging of malignant tumours of the long bones in children: monitoring response to neoadjuvant chemotherapy and preoperative assessment. Pediatr Radiol 2004;34(8):595–605.

[33] Fletcher BD, Hanna SL, Fairclough DL, et al. Pediatric musculoskeletal tumors: use of dynamic, contrast-enhanced MR imaging to monitor response to chemotherapy. Radiology 1992;184(1): 243–8.

[34] Reddick WE, Wang S, Xiong X, et al. Dynamic magnetic resonance imaging of regional contrast access as an additional prognostic factor in pediatric osteosarcoma. Cancer 2001;91(12):2230–7.

[35] Nakanishi K, Araki N, Yoshikawa H, et al. Alveolar soft part sarcoma. Eur Radiol 1998; 8(5):813–6.

[36] Shapeero LG, Vanel D, Verstraete KL, et al. Fast magnetic resonance imaging with contrast for soft tissue sarcoma viability. Clin Orthop 2002;(397):212–27.

[37] van Rijswijk CS, Geirnaerdt MJ, Hogendoorn PC, et al. Dynamic contrast-enhanced MR imaging in monitoring response to isolated limb perfusion in high-grade soft tissue sarcoma: initial results. Eur Radiol 2003;13(8):1849–58.

[38] Vanel D, Bonvalot S, Guinebretiere JM, et al. MR imaging in the evaluation of isolated limb perfusion: a prospective study of 18 cases. Skeletal Radiol 2004;33(3):150–6.

[39] Sijens PE. Phosphorus MR spectroscopy in the treatment of human extremity sarcomas. NMR Biomed 1998;11(7):341–53.

[40] Sostman HD, Prescott DM, Dewhirst MW, et al. MR imaging and spectroscopy for prognostic evaluation in soft-tissue sarcomas. Radiology 1994;190(1):269–75.

[41] Kettelhack C, Wickede M, Vogl T, et al. 31Phosphorus-magnetic resonance spectroscopy to assess histologic tumor response noninvasively after isolated limb perfusion for soft tissue tumors. Cancer 2002;94(5):1557–64.

[42] Redmond OM, Stack JP, O'Connor NG, et al. 31P MRS as an early prognostic indicator of patient response to chemotherapy. Magn Reson Med 1992;25(1):30–44.

[43] Koutcher JA, Ballon D, Graham M, et al. 31P NMR spectra of extremity sarcomas: diversity of metabolic profiles and changes in response to chemotherapy. Magn Reson Med 1990;16(1): 19–34.

[44] Sijens PE, Eggermont AM, van Dijk PV, et al. 31P magnetic resonance spectroscopy as predictor of clinical response in human extremity sarcomas treated by single dose TNF-alpha + melphalan isolated limb perfusion. NMR Biomed 1995;8(5):215–24.

[45] Choong PF, Nizam I, Ngan SY, et al. Thallium-201 scintigraphy–a predictor of tumour necrosis in soft tissue sarcoma following preoperative radiotherapy? Eur J Surg Oncol 2003; 29(10):908–15.

[46] Menendez LR, Fideler BM, Mirra J. Thallium-201 scanning for the evaluation of osteosarcoma and soft-tissue sarcoma. A study of the evaluation and predictability of the histological response to chemotherapy. J Bone Joint Surg Am 1993;75(4):526–31.

[47] Demetri GD, von Mehren M, Blanke CD, et al. Efficacy and safety of imatinib mesylate in advanced gastrointestinal stromal tumors. N Engl J Med 2002;347(7):472–80.

[48] Verweij J, Casali PG, Zalcberg J, et al. Progression-free survival in gastrointestinal stromal tumours with high-dose imatinib: randomised trial. Lancet 2004;364(9440):1127–34.

[49] Joensuu H, Roberts PJ, Sarlomo-Rikala M, et al. Effect of the tyrosine kinase inhibitor STI571 in a patient with a metastatic gastrointestinal stromal tumor. N Engl J Med 2001;344(14): 1052–6.

[50] Gayed I, Vu T, Iyer R, et al. The role of 18F-FDG PET in staging and early prediction of response to therapy of recurrent gastrointestinal stromal tumors. J Nucl Med 2004;45(1):17–21.

[51] Goerres GW, Stupp R, Barghouth G, et al. The value of PET, CT and in-line PET/CT in patients with gastrointestinal stromal tumours: long-term outcome of treatment with imatinib mesylate. Eur J Nucl Med Mol Imaging 2005;32(2):153–62.

[52] Jager PL, Gietema JA, van der Graaf WT. Imatinib mesylate for the treatment of gastrointestinal stromal tumours: best monitored with FDG PET. Nucl Med Commun 2004;25(5): 433–8.

[53] Stroobants S, Goeminne J, Seegers M, et al. 18FDG-Positron emission tomography for the early prediction of response in advanced soft tissue sarcoma treated with imatinib mesylate (Glivec). Eur J Cancer 2003;39(14):2012–20.

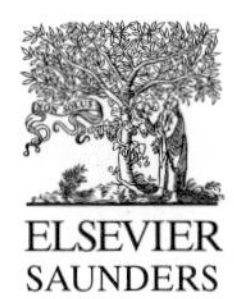
ELSEVIER
SAUNDERS

Hematol Oncol Clin N Am
19 (2005) 489–500

HEMATOLOGY/
ONCOLOGY
CLINICS OF
NORTH AMERICA

Neoadjuvant and Adjuvant Therapy for Extremity Soft Tissue Sarcomas

Michelle Scurr, BMed, FRACP[a,*], Ian Judson, MD, FRCP[a,b]

[a]*Cancer Research-UK Centre for Cancer Therapeutics, Institute of Cancer Research, Sycamore House, Downs Road, Sutton, Surrey SM2 5PT, UK*
[b]*Sarcoma Unit, Mulberry House, Royal Marsden NHS Foundation Trust, Fulham Road, London SW3 6JJ, UK*

Despite the overall good prognosis in patients who have localized soft tissue sarcoma (STS) of the extremities, approximately half of those who have high-risk features ultimately will die from metastatic disease that was present as microscopic foci at the time of diagnosis [1]. The principal role of adjuvant and neoadjuvant chemotherapy is to improve the "cure" rate through eradication of these microscopic foci, and there is good evidence for a survival benefit in other solid tumors groups. Over the last 30 years there have been numerous studies attempting to determine whether adjuvant or neoadjuvant systemic chemotherapy does lead to an improvement in disease-specific survival in patients who have localized STS. Most studies have been too small or had serious flaws in study design and have failed to provide a clear answer. A meta-analysis has shown some benefit for doxorubicin-based chemotherapy with a nonsignificant trend toward improved overall survival in mostly because of a modest but significant survival advantage for those who have extremity STS [2]. It is still unclear whether there may be a role for systemic chemotherapy in patients who have high-risk localized STS of the extremities. This article discusses some of the issues surrounding this most controversial area in the management of STS.

* Corresponding author.
E-mail address: michelle.scurr@icr.ac.uk (M. Scurr).

0889-8588/05/$ – see front matter
doi:10.1016/j.hoc.2005.03.003

Background

Patients who present with localized STS of the extremities have a potentially curable disease, with a 5-year disease-specific survival (DSS) of 76% to 79% [1,3] when complete resection is achieved. However, despite optimal local treatment, approximately 50% of patients who have high-risk features will relapse and die from metastatic disease [1]. These patients have occult systemic disease at the time of presentation, which will gradually become clinically apparent. Once macroscopic metastatic disease is evident the outlook is poor, with a median survival of only 11.7 months [4]. This fact has led to an intensive investigation of adjuvant and neoadjuvant systemic therapy in localized STS over the last 30 years.

Adjuvant and neoadjuvant chemotherapy are used to eradicate occult metastatic disease, and are based on the same principals: smaller tumors have a higher growth fraction and are thus potentially more chemosensitive [5]; and the larger a tumor becomes, the more likely it is that a chemoresistant clone will spontaneously arise [6]. Adjuvant chemotherapy allows for immediate treatment of the local disease; however, this means that treatment of potential metastatic disease is delayed until recovery from surgery. Another potential problem with adjuvant chemotherapy is that, unlike neoadjuvant therapy, it is not possible to determine the sensitivity of the sarcoma to the particular chemotherapy regimen. Some evidence suggests that the response of the sarcoma to neoadjuvant therapy may also have prognostic value for survival [7,8], although this is not certain, with some studies showing no association [9]. A further advantage for neoadjuvant chemotherapy is that it allows for immediate treatment of potential occult disease, although this is counterbalanced by the potentially deleterious delay in definitive local treatment.

The principal aim of adjuvant or neoadjuvant chemotherapy is to improve the cure rate in patients who have localized STS, which requires that a clinically significant improvement in DSS or overall survival (OS) be demonstrated consistently. For some solid tumors, such as breast cancer [10] and colorectal cancer [11], a role for adjuvant chemotherapy as manifest by an improved overall survival has certainly been demonstrated. However, the role for systemic treatment in the management of localized STS is unclear, as is discussed later. Some evidence supports adjuvant chemotherapy in patients who have high-risk localized STS of the extremities, but this is still controversial. The remainder of this article discusses some of the issues surrounding this controversial area of STS management.

Prognostic variables

Three quarters of all patients who have localized extremity STS will not relapse after optimal local treatment and therefore do not need any further treatment to be cured. It is important to limit treatment to those most at risk for relapse. There are several reasons why it is important to limit treatment to those most at risk for relapse; the most important is to avoid unnecessarily exposing already "cured" patients to the serious and even potentially fatal toxicities associated with systemic chemotherapy. Conversely, it is also important to be able to identify those patients who are most likely to relapse, as these patients will not be cured unless the microscopic disease is eradicated. It is not yet possible to determine on an individual basis which patient has microscopic foci of disease and is therefore most likely to benefit; however, validated prognostic variables can identify those groups of patients who are most at risk.

There have been several studies, mostly retrospective reviews from single institutions, evaluating prognostic factors predictive of metastatic relapse and of DSS in localized STS of extremities. The factors predictive of metastatic recurrence are essentially the same as those predictive of poorer disease specific survival. The most important and influential prognostic variable for metastatic recurrence and DSS is grade [1,3,12–21]. The two other variables that have consistently demonstrated significant influence are those of size of primary tumor and depth of the tumor in relation to the investing fascia [1,3,12–18,20,21]. Thus, the American Joint Committee on Cancer and the International Union Against Cancer have incorporated these three factors into the validated TNM staging system for STS [22].

One of the largest studies analyzed prospectively collected data on 1041 adult patients who had localized extremity STS (stage IA to IIIB) treated at a single institution between 1982 and 1994 [13]. Factors predictive for metastatic relapse were high tumor grade, primary tumor size larger than10 cm, deep location, recurrent local disease at presentation, and leiomyosarcoma. Grade was found to most strongly predict DSS with a relative risk of 4.0 (95% CI, 2.5–6.6), although its importance in predicting survival gradually decreased. Other independently predictive factors of DSS included primary tumor size larger than 5 cm, deep location, positive microscopic margins, leiomyosarcoma, or malignant peripheral nerve sheath tumor histology. These results are similar to a more recently published review of more than 1200 patients who had completely excised localized STS of the extremities treated at a single institution between 1992 and 2001 [3]. As expected, grade, size, and depth of the tumor were found to independently predict distant recurrence-free survival and DSS. As in the earlier study [13] and others [1,17], positive microscopic surgical margins were associated with a poorer DSS. However, other studies have not found the surgical margin to be a significant variable for survival in localized STS of the extremities [12,18,19]. Proximal lesions were found to have a statistically significant worse DSS than those with distal extremity lesions as seen in other studies, and may be reflective of many variables, including larger size of proximal lesions [3,17]. No difference in survival was seen between those patients who had upper extremity lesions and those who had lower extremity lesions in this cohort of patients; however, some studies have shown a higher metastatic rate or poorer survival for those patients who have lower extremity STS [13–16].

Grade, size, and depth are the three most important and consistent independent variables for DSS, and several studies have shown a continuum of decreasing survival with higher grade and larger tumors. In a study by Stojadinovic et al [1], the 5-year DSS for patients who had a small ($\leq$5 cm) low-grade extremity tumor was 98%, and 8% for those who had a small ($\leq$5 cm) high-grade tumor. In patients who had a large (>10 cm) high-grade tumor, the DSS was only 50%. Based on these known variables and on the influence more than one high-risk factor can have on survival, Kattan et al [23] constructed a nomogram for predicting 12-year sarcoma survival that has recently been validated [24]. Therefore, the patients most likely to benefit from effective systemic treatment are those who have high-grade, large, and deep STS. There may be a role for those patients who have microscopically positive surgical margins, but this remains to be shown [23–25].

Adjuvant chemotherapy

Only doxorubicin and ifosfamide have been shown to have significant clinical activity as single agents in STS. Doxorubicin is regarded as the most active single agent, with reported response rates of approximately 25% [26–28], although more recent studies have reported response rates as low as 9% [29]. Two other anthracyclines, epirubicin [28,30] and liposomal doxorubicin [29], have shown activity but with no advantage over standard doxorubicin. Single-agent ifosfamide has been shown to have similar response rates to doxorubicin, with objective responses in the range of 20% to 30% [31–33]. In the metastatic setting, the combination of doxorubicin and ifosfamide has proven to be tolerable, with higher response rates than seen with the drugs given as single agents, but with no survival advantage and higher toxicity [34,35]. Dacarbazine has shown modest activity [36], but most other agents have shown limited or no clinical activity in this group of tumors.

Over the years there have been several randomized trials investigating the role of doxorubicin-based adjuvant chemotherapy in localized STS, with doxorubicin being used either as a single agent or as part of a combination regimen. For most of the studies there is heterogeneity in the anatomic sites, with most including a cohort of extremity tumors. However, five trials have been published that have concentrated on extremity STS [37–43], although one is not strictly adjuvant as all patients received intra-arterial doxorubicin preoperatively [43]. In this study, patients who had high-grade extremity STS were randomized postoperatively to high-dose doxorubicin (90 mg/m^2) or observation, and at a median follow-up of 30 months there was no benefit seen for DSS or OS with the addition of adjuvant doxorubicin. Picci et al [37] also randomized patients who had high-grade extremity tumors to either single-agent doxorubicin postsurgical treatment or no chemotherapy. However, in this study a significant improvement in the 5-year disease-free survival (DFS) and the

5-year OS was seen in the cohort treated with adjuvant chemotherapy ($P < .05$). Benjamin et al [38] reported a randomized study in patients who had truncal or extremity STS in which the chemotherapeutic regimen consisted of doxorubicin, vincristine, cyclophosphamide, and dactinomycin. In the group of 46 patients who had extremity STS and a median follow-up time of more than 10 years, there was evidence for improved relapse-free survival ($P = .04$) but not for OS. The National Cancer Institute randomized patients who had high-grade extremity tumors to postoperative combination chemotherapy (doxorubicin, cyclophosphamide, and high-dose methotrexate) or no chemotherapy [39,40]. An early analysis [39] at a median follow-up of 1.9 years reported a significant benefit for DFS ($P = .008$) and OS ($P = .04$), but at a median follow-up of 7.1 years, the advantage for OS was lost [39].

In addition, many patients who have extremity STS have been included in randomized adjuvant studies where there was no restriction in the anatomic site of the primary disease. Some have used single-agent doxorubicin [44–46] with no significant survival advantage seen for adjuvant treatment. Several studies have used combination regimens and again have provided no clear answer. The European Organization for Research and Treatment of Cancer (EORTC) randomized 468 patients to either a combination regimen consisting of cyclophosphamide, vincristine, doxorubicin, and DTIC (CYVADIC) or observation alone [47] and found no significant improvement in overall survival. A significant improvement was seen for relapse-free survival and local recurrence rate, but this was limited to the group of trunk and head and neck tumors and was not seen for STS of the extremities. Fondation Bergonié also compared CYVADIC regimen with no chemotherapy in 65 patients, but in contrast to the EORTC, found that the regimen improved 5-year OS ($P = .002$) [48]. The Mayo Clinic randomized 76 patients (48 patients who had extremity STS) to no chemotherapy or to a complicated multidrug regimen that included a low dose of doxorubicin (total cumulative dose, 200 mg/m^2) and found no statistical evidence of improved survival with the regimen [49].

It is difficult to draw any conclusions regarding the role for adjuvant chemotherapy in localized extremity STS from the individual trials, as not only are the outcomes often contradictory but there are serious flaws in the design of many of the studies, diminishing the ability to make meaningful interpretations of the results. The sample size for many of the studies were too small to allow proper statistical analysis, ineligibility rates were high in several studies, and patients at low risk for relapse (low grade, small size) were included in some studies, potentially diminishing the power of the studies to show any advantage for chemotherapy for those at greatest risk for relapse. The use of the other agents in the combination regimens is important, as most have limited or no activity as single agents in advanced STS and thus would only have served to increase toxicity. Several meta-analyses have been published trying to assess the potential role of adjuvant chemotherapy in localized STS [2,50–52]. The first three meta-analyses were literature-based (where the analysis is based on the published results) and included only published studies, with Zalupski et al [51] concentrating on STS of the extremities. All three meta-analyses found that adjuvant chemotherapy significantly improved OS. There are many potential biases inherent in the design of these meta-analyses, including publication bias, inappropriate patient exclusions, variable follow-up times, and single/fixed time-point endpoint analyses. In an attempt to minimize the effect of these biases, a multinational working party, the Sarcoma Meta-analysis Collaboration, performed a quantitative meta-analysis of all published and unpublished randomized studies of adjuvant doxorubicin-based chemotherapy versus no chemotherapy that had completed accrual before December 1992 [2]. The analysis used updated individual patient data, which allowed a more accurate determination of clinically relevant endpoints, including times to first local recurrence and metastatic recurrence, DFS and overall survival, and allowing subgroup analyses to be performed. Thirteen published studies and one unpublished study were identified and are comprised of 1568 patients. Doxorubicin doses ranged from 50 to 90 mg/m^2 per cycle (planned cumulative doses, 200–550 mg/m^2), given as a single agent in six studies and in combination in the other eight studies; only the small unpublished study from the Swiss Group for Clinical Cancer Research included ifosfamide. Adjuvant chemotherapy was found to significantly improve local control ($P = .016$) with a 27% reduction in the risk for local recurrence. There was also a highly significant benefit seen with adjuvant chemotherapy for distant recurrence-free interval ($P = .003$) and in overall recurrence-free survival ($P = .001$). For the primary endpoint of OS, which is the principal outcome required for adjuvant therapy to be effective, there was a trend in favor of chemotherapy (hazard ratio 0.89 [95% CI, 0.73–1.06]), but this did not reach statistical significance ($P = .12$), representing a potential absolute benefit of 4% at 10 years. There was no advantage for combination chemotherapy over single-agent doxorubicin, although this result must be interpreted with caution as ifosfamide was only used in one small study, most of the agents in the combination regimens have shown limited or no activity in STS as single agents, and doses in some studies were substandard. In a subset analysis of the patients who had extremity STS (n = 886), adjuvant chemotherapy was associated with an improved overall survival (hazard ratio 0.8, $P = .029$), which equated to a potential 7% absolute improvement at 10 years. However, there was no clear evidence that the results for other sites were any different from those for extremity STS ($P = .58$).

Since the publication of this meta-analysis, three randomized studies have been published that evaluated the combination of ifosfamide with an anthracycline in the adjuvant setting compared with no chemotherapy [41,42,53,54], with one study confined to STS of the extremities [41,42]. The Austrian Cooperative Soft Tissue Sarcoma group [53] reported a study in which 59 patients who had high-risk localized STS, defined as grade 2 and larger than 5 cm in size, or grade 3 and any size, were randomized to an intensified combination chemotherapy regimen comprising ifosfamide, dacarbazine, and doxorubicin given every 14 days with granulocyte-colony stimulating factor (G-CSF) support, or to no chemotherapy after surgery. There was no survival benefit seen and the study closed early because of poor accrual. Petrioli et al [54] recently reported on 88 patients who had grade 2 or 3 STS randomized to chemotherapy or observation after surgery. Patients randomized to chemotherapy between 1985 and 1991 (n = 26) received single-agent epirubicin, and those randomized to chemotherapy between 1991 and 1996 (n = 19) received epirubicin and ifosfamide. There was an improved 5-year DFS ($P = .01$) and a trend toward improved 5-year OS ($P = .06$) for those patients randomized to adjuvant chemotherapy. When the results were stratified according to whether the patients received ifosfamide in addition to epirubicin, there was a significant advantage seen for the addition of ifosfamide, with significant DFS ($P = .008$) and OS ($P = .01$) when compared with the control group from the same accrual period; no advantage was seen for the subgroup that received single-agent epirubicin over the control group from the same accrual period. These results need to be interpreted with caution given the small numbers in each of the treatment arms. Frustaci et al [41] randomized patients who had high-risk (high grade and size ≥5 cm) STS of the extremities to ifosfamide and epirubicin or to no chemotherapy. The planned accrual was initially 190 patients, but the trial closed early (104 patients), as an interim analysis demonstrated a significant DFS advantage ($P = .001$) for those randomized to adjuvant chemotherapy. At a median follow-up of 59 months there was a significant improvement in median DFS seen for those patients in the treatment arm compared with the control arm (48 months versus 16 months, respectively, $P = .04$), and median OS (75 months versus 46 months respectively, $P = .03$). However, a recent update with a longer follow-up (89.6 months) has reported that although there is still a difference in OS in an intention-to-treat analysis, it is no longer statistically significant [42].

The EORTC has recently closed to accrual an adjuvant trial for high-grade soft tissue sarcomas using doxorubicin 7 5mg/m^2 and ifosfamide 5 g/m^2 with G-CSF support. Although this study is not confined to patients who have extremity STS, it is hoped that the results of this study will help determine the role of adjuvant chemotherapy, but it will take several years before any meaningful results will be available.

Neoadjuvant chemotherapy

The data relating to the role of neoadjuvant chemotherapy in improving survival in patients who have localized STS of the extremities is limited, with most deriving from retrospective analyses of small patient sample size.

There has been only one randomized study of neoadjuvant chemotherapy in localized STS [55]. This multinational phase 2 study compared neoadjuvant ifosfamide and doxorubicin with surgery alone for high-risk, potentially resectable STS of all anatomic sites. "High-risk" was defined as any of the following: tumor 8 cm or larger of any grade, grade 2/3 tumors smaller than 8 cm, grade 2/3 locally recurrent tumors, or grade 2/3 tumors with inadequate surgery performed in the previous 6 weeks and requiring further surgery. The study randomized 67 eligible patients to neoadjuvant treatment and 67 eligible patients to surgery alone. The study was initially designed as a phase 2/3 study but was closed after completion of the phase 2 part because of slow accrual. Although the study was not adequately powered to determine a survival benefit, neoadjuvant chemotherapy did not demonstrate any survival advantage over no chemotherapy, with similar 5-year DFS and OS: 56% versus 52% ($P = .35$) and 65% versus 64%, respectively.

Several retrospective analyses have suggested a survival advantage for the use of neoadjuvant chemotherapy in patients who have high-risk feature. DeLaney et al [56] performed a nonrandomized study using preoperative and postoperative chemotherapy with interdigitated radiotherapy and compared the patients with historical case controls who were not treated with chemotherapy. Chemotherapy consisted of doxorubicin, ifosfamide, and dacarbazine and was given for three cycles preoperatively and three cycles postoperatively, with radiotherapy between each preoperative chemotherapy to a dose of 44 Gy, and then 16 Gy given before adjuvant chemotherapy. There was no difference in local control; however, significant improvements were seen for 5-year metastasis-free survival (75% versus 44%, $P = .016$), DFS (70% versus 42%, $P = .002$), and OS (87% versus 58%, $P = .003$) for those patients who were treated with the chemoradiation compared with the historical controls. Grobmyer et al [57] performed a retrospective cohort study comparing neoadjuvant doxorubicin and ifosfamide in 74 patients who had localized high-grade, deep, larger than 5 cm STS of the extremities with 282 patients treated with surgery alone. The patients who were treated with neoadjuvant chemotherapy were younger (median age of 50 years) than those treated by surgery alone (median age of 62 years), and had larger tumors (12 cm versus 10 cm, respectively). The overall 3-year DSS was 73% (95% CI, 68%–78%), with those patients who received neoadjuvant chemotherapy having a significantly better DSS ($P = .02$). After stratification for risk factors, this benefit appeared to be limited to those who had tumors larger than 10 cm, with those treated by surgery alone having a 3-year DSS of 62% and those treated with neoadjuvant chemotherapy a 3-year DSS of 83%, representing a 21% survival benefit. A small retrospective study evaluating radiographic response to neoadjuvant chemotherapy in patients who had stage II or III STS (42 extremity, 23 retroperitoneal) found that the patients receiving an ifosfamide-containing regimen had a higher percentage of response ($P = .094$), and that radiographic response was associated with a significant improvement in OS compared with those patients who had stable disease or progressive disease by radiographic criteria [8]. Other retrospective studies have suggested a survival advantage for patients who respond to neoadjuvant chemotherapy [7,58], although a study by Pisters et al [9] demonstrated no improvement in OS in those patients who had stage IIIB STS of the extremities treated with neoadjuvant doxorubicin-based chemotherapy.

Two retrospective reviews have recently been published evaluating the role of chemotherapy in patients who have high-risk extremity STS [59,60]. Cormier et al [59] reported an observational study of 674 patients presenting with localized high-risk extremity STS at two institutions from 1984 until June 1999. Overall, 336 patients (50%) received chemotherapy and of these, 64% received preoperative chemotherapy and 35% postoperative chemotherapy. Doxorubicin was used either alone or in combination in 88% of cases. Patients who were treated with chemotherapy were significantly younger than those who did not receive treatment ($P<.001$). There was an interesting time-varying effect seen with the chemotherapy for survival endpoints. Patients treated with chemotherapy had a lower risk for dying during the first year, but this risk increased sharply; conversely, those who did not receive chemotherapy were initially at a higher risk for dying of sarcoma, but this risk decreased markedly during the next 2 years, so that after 1 year a patient who had received chemotherapy had a higher risk for dying of sarcoma than those who did not receive chemotherapy at all. This pattern was seen for distant recurrence-free interval, distant DFS, overall DFS, and DSS. Eilber et al [60] analyzed 245 patients who had high-grade, large, localized liposarcoma of the extremities. Patients were treated with a doxorubicin-based regimen (34%), an ifosfamide-based regimen (26%), or no chemotherapy (40%). There was no difference for 5-year DSS seen in those treated with doxorubicin compared with a contemporary cohort of patients who received no chemotherapy, whereas a statistically significant improvement was seen for those treated with ifosfamide compared with no chemotherapy (92% versus 65%, $P=.003$).

Summary

Despite three decades of extensive research we still have no clear answer as to whether adjuvant/neoadjuvant chemotherapy can improve survival in patients who have localized STS of the extremities, although the evidence seems to suggest that it may afford a modest improvement in survival in those patients who have high-risk features. Why has it taken so long and so many studies to reach this stage of ongoing uncertainty? There are many reasons. First, most of the studies have been too small to demonstrate a significant survival benefit. Secondly, patients have been included who have low-risk features (diluting any effect of the chemotherapy). Most importantly, patients have been treated with either substandard doses of effective agents or combinations of agents known to have little to no activity in this tumor group. Furthermore, there are few chemotherapeutic agents with any significant activity against STS, and unless the results from the recently closed EORTC study show otherwise, any benefit will be modest at best. It may be that innovative combinations with antiangiogenic agents or signal transduction inhibitors in addition to traditional chemotherapy can improve the "cure" rate that has not changed in at least the last 20 years [3].

References

[1] Stojadinovic A, Leung DH, Allen P, et al. Primary adult soft tissue sarcoma: time-dependent influence of prognostic variables. J Clin Oncol 2002;20(21):4344–52.

[2] Sarcoma Meta-analysis Collaboration. Adjuvant chemotherapy for localised resectable soft-tissue sarcoma of adults: meta-analysis of individual data. Lancet 1997;350(9092):1647–54.

[3] Weitz J, Antonescu CR, Brennan MF. Localized extremity soft tissue sarcoma: improved knowledge with unchanged survival over time. J Clin Oncol 2003;21(14):2719–25.

[4] Greenlee RT, Hill-Harmon MB, Murray T, et al. Cancer statistics, 2001. CA Cancer J Clin 2001;51(1):15–36.

[5] Norton L. Adjuvant breast cancer therapy: current status and future strategies–growth kinetics and the improved drug therapy of breast cancer. Semin Oncol 1999;26(1 Suppl 3):1–4.

[6] Goldie JH, Coldman AJ. A mathematic model for relating the drug sensitivity of tumors to their spontaneous mutation rate. Cancer Treat Rep 1979;63(11–12):1727–33.

[7] Eilber FC, Rosen G, Eckardt J, et al. Treatment-induced pathologic necrosis: a predictor of local recurrence and survival in patients receiving neoadjuvant therapy for high-grade extremity soft tissue sarcomas. J Clin Oncol 2001;19(13):3203–9.

[8] Meric F, Hess KR, Varma DG, et al. Radiographic response to neoadjuvant chemotherapy is a predictor of local control and survival in soft tissue sarcomas. Cancer 2002;95(5):1120–6.

[9] Pisters PW, Patel SR, Varma DG, et al. Preoperative chemotherapy for stage IIIB extremity soft tissue sarcoma: long-term results from a single institution. J Clin Oncol 1997;15(12): 3481–7.

[10] Early Breast Cancer Trialists' Collaborative Group. Polychemotherapy for early breast cancer: an overview of the randomised trials. Lancet 1998;352(9132):930–42.

[11] Moertel CG, Fleming TR, Macdonald JS, et al. Fluorouracil plus levamisole as effective adjuvant therapy after resection of stage III colon carcinoma: a final report. Ann Intern Med 1995; 122(5):321–6.

[12] Trovik CS, Bauer HC, Alvegard TA, et al. Surgical margins, local recurrence and metastasis in soft tissue sarcomas: 559 surgically-treated patients from the Scandinavian Sarcoma Group Register. Eur J Cancer 2000;36(6):710–6.

[13] Pisters PW, Leung DH, Woodruff J, et al. Analysis of prognostic factors in 1,041 patients with localized soft tissue sarcomas of the extremities. J Clin Oncol 1996;14(5):1679–89.

[14] Zagars GK, Ballo MT, Pisters PW, et al. Prognostic factors for patients with localized soft-tissue sarcoma treated with conservation surgery and radiation therapy: an analysis of 225 patients. Cancer 2003;97(10):2530–43.

[15] Gerrand CH, Bell RS, Wunder JS, et al. The influence of anatomic location on outcome in patients with soft tissue sarcoma of the extremity. Cancer 2003;97(2):485–92.

[16] Vraa S, Keller J, Nielsen OS, et al. Prognostic factors in soft tissue sarcomas: the Aarhus experience. Eur J Cancer 1998;34(12):1876–82.

[17] Collin C, Godbold J, Hajdu S, et al. Localized extremity soft tissue sarcoma: an analysis of factors affecting survival. J Clin Oncol 1987;5(4):601–12.

[18] Gaynor JJ, Tan CC, Casper ES, et al. Refinement of clinicopathologic staging for localized soft tissue sarcoma of the extremity: a study of 423 adults. J Clin Oncol 1992;10(8):1317–29.

[19] Vraa S, Keller J, Nielsen OS, et al. Soft-tissue sarcoma of the thigh: surgical margin influences local recurrence but not survival in 152 patients. Acta Orthop Scand 2001;72(1):72–7.

[20] McKee MD, Liu DF, Brooks JJ, et al. The prognostic significance of margin width for extremity and trunk sarcoma. J Surg Oncol 2004;85(2):68–76.

[21] Stotter AT, A'Hern RP, Fisher C, et al. The influence of local recurrence of extremity soft tissue sarcoma on metastasis and survival. Cancer 1990;65(5):1119–29.

[22] American Joint Committee on Cancer. Cancer staging manual. 6th edition. New York: Springer; 2002.

[23] Kattan MW, Leung DH, Brennan MF. Postoperative nomogram for 12-year sarcoma-specific death. J Clin Oncol 2002;20(3):791–6.

[24] Eilber FC, Brennan MF, Eilber FR, et al. Validation of the postoperative nomogram for 12-year sarcoma-specific mortality. Cancer 2004;101(10):2270–5.

[25] Fleming JB, Berman RS, Cheng SC, et al. Long-term outcome of patients with American Joint Committee on Cancer stage IIB extremity soft tissue sarcomas. J Clin Oncol 1999;17(9): 2772–80.

[26] Bramwell VH, Mouridsen HT, Mulder JH, et al. Carminomycin vs adriamycin in advanced soft tissue sarcomas: an EORTC randomised phase II study. Eur J Cancer Clin Oncol 1983;19(8): 1097–104.

[27] Borden EC, Amato DA, Rosenbaum C, et al. Randomized comparison of three adriamycin regimens for metastatic soft tissue sarcomas. J Clin Oncol 1987;5(6):840–50.

[28] Mouridsen HT, Bastholt L, Somers R, et al. Adriamycin versus epirubicin in advanced soft tissue sarcomas. A randomized phase II/phase III study of the EORTC Soft Tissue and Bone Sarcoma Group. Eur J Cancer Clin Oncol 1987;23(10):1477–83.

[29] Judson I, Radford JA, Harris M, et al. Randomised phase II trial of pegylated liposomal doxorubicin (DOXIL/CAELYX) versus doxorubicin in the treatment of advanced or metastatic soft tissue sarcoma: a study by the EORTC Soft Tissue and Bone Sarcoma Group. Eur J Cancer 2001;37(7):870–7.

[30] Nielsen OS, Dombernowsky P, Mouridsen H, et al. High-dose epirubicin is not an alternative to standard-dose doxorubicin in the treatment of advanced soft tissue sarcomas. A study of the EORTC soft tissue and bone sarcoma group. Br J Cancer 1998;78(12):1634–9.

[31] Antman KH, Ryan L, Elias A, et al. Response to ifosfamide and mesna: 124 previously treated patients with metastatic or unresectable sarcoma. J Clin Oncol 1989;7(1):126–31.

[32] Bramwell VH, Mouridsen HT, Santoro A, et al. Cyclophosphamide versus ifosfamide: a randomized phase II trial in adult soft-tissue sarcomas. The European Organization for Research and Treatment of Cancer [EORTC], Soft Tissue and Bone Sarcoma Group. Cancer Chemother Pharmacol 1993;31(Suppl 2):S180–4.

[33] Benjamin RS, Legha SS, Patel SR, et al. Single-agent ifosfamide studies in sarcomas of soft tissue and bone: the M.D. Anderson experience. Cancer Chemother Pharmacol 1993; 31(Suppl 2):S174–9.

[34] Edmonson JH, Ryan LM, Blum RH, et al. Randomized comparison of doxorubicin alone versus ifosfamide plus doxorubicin or mitomycin, doxorubicin, and cisplatin against advanced soft tissue sarcomas. J Clin Oncol 1993;11(7):1269–75.

[35] Le Cesne A, Judson I, Crowther D, et al. Randomized phase III study comparing conventional-dose doxorubicin plus ifosfamide versus high-dose doxorubicin plus ifosfamide plus recombinant human granulocyte-macrophage colony-stimulating factor in advanced soft tissue sarcomas: a trial of the European Organization for Research and Treatment of Cancer/Soft Tissue and Bone Sarcoma Group. J Clin Oncol 2000;18(14):2676–84.

[36] Gottlieb JA, Benjamin RS, Baker LH, et al. Role of DTIC (NSC-45388) in the chemotherapy of sarcomas. Cancer Treat Rep 1976;60(2):199–203.

[37] Picci P, Bacci G, Gherlinzoni F, et al. Results of randomized trial for the treatment of localized soft tissue tumors (STS) of the extremities in adult patients. In: Ryan JR, Baker LH, editors. Recent concepts in sarcoma treatment. Dordrecht (The Netherlands): Kluwer Academic Publishers; 1988. p. 144–8.

[38] Benjamin RS, Terjanian TO, Fenoglio CJ, et al. The importance of combination chemotherapy for adjuvant treatment of high-risk patients with soft- tissue sarcomas of the extremities. In: Salmon SE, editor. Adjuvant therapy of cancer V. Orlando (FL): Grune and Stratton; 1987. p. 735–44.

[39] Rosenberg SA, Tepper J, Glatstein E, et al. Prospective randomized evaluation of adjuvant chemotherapy in adults with soft tissue sarcomas of the extremities. Cancer 1983;52(3): 424–34.

[40] Chang AE, Kinsella T, Glatstein E, et al. Adjuvant chemotherapy for patients with high-grade soft-tissue sarcomas of the extremity. J Clin Oncol 1988;6(9):1491–500.

[41] Frustaci S, Gherlinzoni F, De Paoli A, et al. Adjuvant chemotherapy for adult soft tissue

sarcomas of the extremities and girdles: results of the Italian randomized cooperative trial. J Clin Oncol 2001;19(5):1238–47.

[42] Frustaci S, De Paoli A, Bidoli E, et al. Ifosfamide in the adjuvant therapy of soft tissue sarcomas. Oncology 2003;65(Suppl 2):80–4.

[43] Eilber FR, Giuliano AE, Huth JF, et al. A randomized prospective trial using postoperative adjuvant chemotherapy (adriamycin) in high-grade extremity soft-tissue sarcoma. Am J Clin Oncol 1988;11(1):39–45.

[44] Alvegard TA, Sigurdsson H, Mouridsen H, et al. Adjuvant chemotherapy with doxorubicin in high-grade soft tissue sarcoma: a randomized trial of the Scandinavian Sarcoma Group. J Clin Oncol 1989;7(10):1504–13.

[45] Baker LH. Adjuvant therapy for soft tissue sarcomas. In: Ryan JR, Baker LH, editors. Recent concepts in sarcoma treatment. Dordrecht (The Netherlands): Kluwer Academic Publishers; 1988. p. 130–5.

[46] Antman K, Ryan L, Borden E, et al. Pooled results from three randomized adjuvant studies of doxorubicin versus observation in soft tissue sarcoma: 10 year results and review of the literature. In: Salmon SE, editor. Adjuvant therapy of cancer VI. Philadelphia: WB Saunders; 1990. p. 529–43.

[47] Bramwell V, Rouesse J, Steward W, et al. Adjuvant CYVADIC chemotherapy for adult soft tissue sarcoma–reduced local recurrence but no improvement in survival: a study of the European Organization for Research and Treatment of Cancer Soft Tissue and Bone Sarcoma Group. J Clin Oncol 1994;12(6):1137–49.

[48] Ravaud A, Bui NB, Coindre JM, et al. Adjuvant chemotherapy with Cyvadic in high risk soft tissue sarcoma: a randomized prospective trial. In: Salmon SE, editor. Adjuvant therapy of cancer VI. Philadelphia: WB Saunders; 1990. p. 556–66.

[49] Edmonson JH, Fleming TR, Ivins JC, et al. Randomized study of systemic chemotherapy following complete excision of nonosseous sarcomas. J Clin Oncol 1984;2(12):1390–6.

[50] Jones GW, Chouinard M, Patel M. Adjuvant adriamycin (doxorubicin) in adult patients with soft tissue sarcomas: a systematic overview and quantitative meta-analysis. Clin Invest Med 1991; 14(Suppl 19):A772.

[51] Zalupski MM, Ryan JR, Hussein ME, et al. Defining the role of adjuvant chemotherapy for patients with soft tissue sarcoma of the extremities. In: Salmon SE, editor. Adjuvant therapy of cancer VII. Philadelphia: JB Lippincott; 1993. p. 385–92.

[52] Tierney JF, Mosseri V, Stewart LA, et al. Adjuvant chemotherapy for soft-tissue sarcoma: review and meta-analysis of the published results of randomised clinical trials. Br J Cancer 1995; 72(2):469–75.

[53] Brodowicz T, Schameis E, Widder J. Intensified adjuvant IFADIC chemotherapy for adult soft tissue sarcoma: a prospective randomized feasibility trial. Sarcoma 2000;4:151–60.

[54] Petrioli R, Coratti A, Correale P, et al. Adjuvant epirubicin with or without ifosfamide for adult soft-tissue sarcoma. Am J Clin Oncol 2002;25(5):468–73.

[55] Gortzak E, Azzarelli A, Buesa J, et al. A randomised phase II study on neo-adjuvant chemotherapy for 'high-risk' adult soft-tissue sarcoma. Eur J Cancer 2001;37(9):1096–103.

[56] DeLaney TF, Spiro IJ, Suit HD, et al. Neoadjuvant chemotherapy and radiotherapy for large extremity soft-tissue sarcomas. Int J Radiat Oncol Biol Phys 2003;56(4):1117–27.

[57] Grobmyer SR, Maki RG, Demetri GD, et al. Neo-adjuvant chemotherapy for primary high-grade extremity soft tissue sarcoma. Ann Oncol 2004;15(11):1667–72.

[58] Pezzi CM, Pollock RE, Evans HL, et al. Preoperative chemotherapy for soft-tissue sarcomas of the extremities. Ann Surg 1990;211(4):476–81.

[59] Cormier JN, Huang X, Xing Y, et al. Cohort analysis of patients with localized, high-risk, extremity soft tissue sarcoma treated at two cancer centers: chemotherapy-associated outcomes. J Clin Oncol 2004;22(22):4567–74.

[60] Eilber FC, Eilber FR, Eckardt J, et al. The impact of chemotherapy on the survival of patients with high-grade primary extremity liposarcoma. Ann Surg 2004;240(4):686–95.

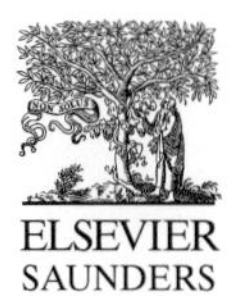

ELSEVIER
SAUNDERS

Hematol Oncol Clin N Am
19 (2005) 501–525

HEMATOLOGY/
ONCOLOGY
CLINICS OF
NORTH AMERICA

Ewing's Sarcoma and Primitive Neuroectodermal Family of Tumors

Richard Carvajal, MD[a], Paul Meyers, MD[b,*]

[a]*Department of Medicine, Memorial Sloan-Kettering Cancer Center, 1275 York Avenue, New York, NY 10021-6007, USA*

[b]*Department of Pediatrics, Memorial Sloan-Kettering Cancer Center, 1275 York Avenue, Room H-1408, New York, NY 10021-6007, USA*

Ewing's sarcoma (ES), first described by James Ewing in 1921 as a diffuse endothelioma of bone, initially was believed to be of perivascular endothelial origin [1]. The Ewing's sarcoma family of tumors (EFT) includes ES of bone (ESB), extraosseous ES (EES), peripheral primitive neuroectodermal tumor of bone (pPNET), and malignant small-cell tumor of the thoracopulmonary region, or Askin's tumor; all of which are now known to be neoplasms of neuroectodermal origin. These tumors are characterized pathologically as small round blue cell tumors, cytogenetically by a t(11;22) or t(21;22) translocation, and molecularly by the presence of chimeric transcripts resulting from the fusion of the EWS gene with genes that encode structurally related transcription factors such as FLI1 or ERG [2].

The degree of neuronal differentiation has been used for histopathologic subclassification of the EFT as classical ES (ESB and EES), which is characterized by minimal evidence of neural differentiation, and pPNET, which displays evidence of neural differentiation by standard microscopy (presence of pseudorosettes), electron microscopy, or immunohistochemistry (two or more neuronal markers, including neuron-specific enolase, Leu-7, or synaptophysin) [3]. Because the behavior, prognosis, and treatment appear to be similar for all subsets of EFT, this histopathologic subclassification may not be clinically significant [4,5], though some debate remains whether neural differentiation predicts for inferior outcome [6,7].

* Corresponding author.
E-mail address: meyersp@mskcc.org (P. Meyers).

doi:10.1016/j.hoc.2005.03.004

Epidemiology and clinical features

ES is the second most common primary malignancy of bone. It is a disease primarily of children and young adults and is rarely seen in older adults. In the United States, approximately 300 cases of ES are diagnosed in children and adolescents under the age of 20 each year. There is a slight male predominance, with an average annual rate of 3.3 per million in men and 2.6 per million in women [8]. The peak incidence in men is between the ages of 10 and 14 years, whereas in women it is between the ages of 5 and 9 years [8]. White children have an approximately ninefold higher incidence rate of ES than black children [9–11]. ES is also uncommon in the Asian patient population [12–14]. The reason for this striking ethnic distribution is not known, although interethnic differences exist for certain alleles of the Ewing's sarcoma (*ews*) gene, which is consistently disrupted in these tumors [15]. Other epidemiologic studies have found limited or inconsistent associations with increased height or weight, age at pubertal growth spurt [9,16–18], paternal occupation in agriculture [19], radiation exposure, or family history of cancer [20,21] and the development of ES. Unlike osteosarcoma, ES is not seen as part of the Li-Fraumeni syndrome [22].

EFT most frequently involves the central axis, occurring in the pelvis in 20% of cases, the chest in 20% of cases, and the head and neck in 9% of cases [23,24]. Bone is the primary site of involvement in 60% of cases. Of this subgroup, 52% are found in the extremities, occurring most frequently in the femur, followed by the tibia, humerus, and fibula [23,24]. Although further subtype analysis is now felt to be highly artificial, historical observations described EES as less common than ESB, with the most common sites of involvement in EES being the trunk (32%), followed by the extremities (26%), head and neck (18%), and retroperitoneum (16%) [25]. Common sites for pPNET include the chest (44%), abdomen and pelvis (26%), extremities (20%), and the head and neck (6%) [26].

Unfavorable clinical prognostic factors in ESB include the presence of fever, anemia [27], elevated serum lactate dehydrogenase (LDH) [28], metastatic disease, and large tumor volume [29,30]. Young children have a better event-free survival (EFS) than older adolescents and adults [27,31–33]. Female sex is a favorable prognostic characteristic [32]. In EFT, distal extremities are the most favorable site; central locations, including the skull, clavicle, vertebrae, ribs, and pelvis, and the proximal extremities, are less favorable [24,27]. The poor prognosis of pelvic tumors is likely associated with the insidious delayed presentation of many of these tumors.

Genetic and molecular characterization

Over 85% of analyzed cases of ES are characterized by a t(11;22)(q24;q12) translocation [2,34–37]. This translocation is also seen in pPNET [38], reflecting the common histogenesis shared with ES. The result of this translocation is the fusion of the *ews* gene, which encodes for an RNA-binding protein of unknown function and is located at 22q12, with the human homolog of the murine *FLI1* gene, a member of the *ETS* family of transcription factors that is located at 11q24 [39]. The chimeric protein product is thought to act as an aberrant transcription factor.

There is significant molecular heterogeneity of the *ews-FLI1* chimeric protein in terms of length and composition resulting from differing combinations of the *ews* and *FLI1* exons. The particular fusion transcript created has been shown to affect the clinical behavior of the tumor. The most common hybrid transcript is formed from the fusion of exon 7 of the *ews* gene with exon 6 of the FLI1 gene and is classified as a type 1 fusion. This transcript has been shown to be associated with a favorable prognosis independent of tumor size, site, or stage [40,41].

Although 90% to 95% of cases involve *FLI1*, less common translocations in EFT have been identified that involve other members of the *ETS* family of transcription factors. These include, in order of frequency, *ERG* (located on chromosome 21) seen in 5% to 10% of cases, *ETV1* (located on chromosome 7), and *E1AF* (located on chromosome 17) [42]. The resulting translocations are t(21;22), t(7;22), and t(17;22) respectively [43].

Secondary cytogenetic alterations have also been found to have prognostic value. For instance, the loss of 16q has been associated with an unfavorable prognosis [44,45]. Recent studies established a correlation between the tumor suppressor gene P53 and the cell proliferation nuclear antigen Ki-67, which were found to be associated with a poorer outcome when present [46]. The most frequent secondary alteration found thus far in EFT is the INK4A deletion. The clinical implications of this genetic marker are still under study [47]. Additional numerical and structural aberrations have been observed in EFTs, also without clear clinical implications. These aberrations include gains of chromosomes 2, 5, 7, 8, 9, and 12, the nonreciprocal translocation t(1;16)(q12;q11.2), and deletion of the short arm of chromosome 1 [48].

Treatment of localized Ewing's sarcoma family of tumors

Before the development of effective chemotherapy, local control measures alone were used for the treatment of localized ESB with 5-year survival rates of 10% to 20% [49–54]. Subclinical metastatic disease is now assumed to be present in nearly all patients because of the significant relapse rate seen in patients who have undergone local treatment without systemic chemotherapy. Micrometastatic disease in the bone marrow has been detected by reverse transcription-polymerase chain reaction (RT-PCR) in 20% to 30% of patients who have apparently localized disease [55–57]. In one retrospective study of patients who had no clinically detectable metastatic disease, the presence of translocation transcripts in the bone marrow detected by RT-PCR was associated with a greater risk for recurrence after treatment [57,58].

The use of adjuvant chemotherapy in EFT began in the early 1970s and has dramatically improved overall survival [59], with 5-year survival rates up to 70% in many large studies and a 10-year EFS of approximately 50% [27,30,32,33, 60–65]. Current treatment strategies for this disease now combine neoadjuvant chemotherapy with surgical resection or radiotherapy followed by adjuvant chemotherapy. The usefulness of neoadjuvant therapy in this disease is suggested by the improved EFS of patients who have minimal or no residual tumor detected on resection compared with those patients who have larger amounts of viable tumor [27,30,31,66,67]. Massive tumor necrosis after induction chemotherapy is a particularly favorable sign [27,68]. In the French Ewing's study (EW88 study), the EFS for patients who had less than 5% viable tumor was 75%, those who had between 5% and 30% was 48%, and those who had greater than 30% viable tumor was 20% [67]. Although the correlation between residual tumor viability and EFS may be because of the addition of neoadjuvant chemotherapy, it is also possible that tumor response to neoadjuvant therapy is simply an indicator of chemosensitivity and that patients who have low residual tumor viability would respond well to adjuvant therapy alone.

Local therapy for Ewing's sarcoma family of tumors

Local therapy initially consisted of radiation therapy or amputation. Radiotherapy to the primary tumor in EFT has resulted in local control rates of up to 90%, particularly for distal extremity lesions. Decreased local control rates were seen with axial lesions and larger lesions. The reported rates of local recurrence, however, were as high as 35% among patients treated with radiation therapy alone [24,62–64,69]. Additionally, significant dose-dependent adverse effects were noted, including growth arrest, pathologic fractures, and radiation-induced sarcomas.

Limb preservation surgery has been performed since the 1970s. With the increased use of limb preservation surgery, a marked decrease in the local relapse rate was noted. Although the local failure rate for nonaxial sites before 1986 was 24%, rates as low as 4% were noted thereafter [27,63,64,70]. For patients who have higher-risk axial disease, the local relapse rate decreased from 31% before 1986 to 15% after 1986. The importance of wide surgical margins in the management of this disease has also become evident over time. In one study of 86 patients who had ES, the 5-year overall survival for those treated with wide or radical resection was 60% versus 40% in those who received marginal or intralesional resection [71].

Some data have suggested improved long-term survival with surgery versus radiotherapy [59,62,72–74], whereas other studies have not shown any significant difference [75,76] or an improvement in local control alone [77]. A study performed at the Rizzoli Orthopaedic Institute that evaluated only patients who had extremity primaries showed that the difference in EFS between patients treated surgically and patients treated by radiotherapy alone was still highly significant in favor of surgery (67% versus 40%, respectively; $P < .001$) [74].

Combined treatment with surgical resection and low-dose radiation has been studied as a means of achieving local control with positive results [32,70,78]. This approach seems to have eliminated the effect of microscopic residual disease on survival [32,79]. Because radiation therapy is known to impair cell turnover and wound healing, a period between surgical resection and the commencement of radiotherapy is important, though the optimal interval has not yet been fully established. In one study of 153 patients who had radiotherapy either before or following postoperative day 60, there was no significant difference in 5-year EFS between the groups, although a trend was noted toward improved local control in those receiving early radiotherapy [80].

Radiotherapy generally is administered in fractionated doses totaling approximately 55.8 Gy to the prechemotherapy tumor volume. The Pediatric Oncology Group (POG) evaluated 40 patients who had ESB between 1983 and 1988 who were randomized to receive involved field radiotherapy totaling 55.8 Gy to the prechemotherapy tumor volume with a 2-cm margin or whole bone irradiation with 39.6 Gy followed by a 16.2-Gy boost [24]. The group noted no difference in local control or EFS. Studies evaluating the utility of hyperfractionated radiation therapy have not shown improved local control or decreased morbidity [81].

With current multimodal protocols that use intensive chemotherapy in addition to local control measures, radiation therapy may approach the degree of local control achieved by surgery [31,32,82,83]. Surgery continues to lead to slightly improved results; however, the fact that smaller, more peripheral lesions that connote lower risk are more likely to be treated surgically may bias this observation.

Systemic therapy in Ewing's sarcoma family of tumors

Cyclophosphamide and doxorubicin are the two most well-studied chemotherapeutic agents in the treatment of EFT. Each was found to produce complete responses in studies performed during the 1960s and early 1970s when used as single agents [84–87]. Vincristine and dactinomycin have also been active and effective in combination with cyclophosphamide [60].

The first Intergroup Ewing Sarcoma Study (IESS-I) performed in the United States between 1973 and 1978 established the importance of using multiagent adjuvant chemotherapy regimens that include alkylating agents and anthracyclines for the treatment of EFT [59]. This study randomized 342 patients to three treatment arms. The first cohort was treated with vincristine, actinomycin D, and cyclophosphamide (VAC), the second was treated with the same combination plus whole lung irradiation (WLI), and the third was treated with vincristine, actinomycin D, cyclophosphamide, and doxorubicin (VACA). The 5-year disease-free survival (DFS) was 24% in the first group, 44% in the second, and 60% in the group treated with doxorubicin.

The second Intergroup Ewing Sarcoma Study (IESS-II) performed between 1978 and 1982 randomized 214 patients to receive either a regimen consisting of high-dose intermittent VACA or one using moderate-dose, continuous VACA as used in IESS-I. A significant difference in 5-year DFS was noted in favor of high- dose intermittent therapy (68% versus 48%; *P*=.02) [75]. This result provided evidence supporting the concept of early aggressive cytoreduction.

Because the Intergroup Ewing Sarcoma Studies demonstrated improved outcomes with the inclusion of doxorubicin, the standard of care for the treatment of EFT became local control measures in combination with multiagent chemotherapy using various schedules and doses of doxorubicin, cyclophosphamide, and vincristine, with or without dactinomycin.

Several important trials have confirmed the efficacy of doxorubicin in this disease. These studies have additionally established large size, pelvic location, and poor histologic response to neoadjuvant chemotherapy as adverse prognostic factors. The ES-79 study performed at St. Jude Children's Research Hospital (SJCRH) between 1978 and 1986 treated 52 patients who had VACA and resulted in a 5-year DFS of 82% in patients who had a tumor less than 8 cm in maximum dimension and 64% in patients who had larger tumors [88]. The first national Ewing's Tumour Study (ET-1), performed in the United Kingdom under the auspices of the United Kingdom Children's Cancer Study Group (UKCCSG) and the Medical Research Council Bone Sarcoma Working Party from 1978 to 1986, evaluated 120 patients who had localized disease treated with VACA [69]. The overall 5-year DFS was 36%. The 5-year DFS by location of tumor was 52% for extremity tumors, 38% for axial tumors, and 13% for pelvic tumors. The German multi-institutional Cooperative Ewing's Sarcoma Study-81 (CESS-81) performed between 1981 and 1985 evaluated 93 patients treated with VACA and resulted in a 5-year DFS of 54% [62]. In patients who had tumor volumes measuring less than 100 mL, the 5-year DFS was 80%. With larger tumor volumes, the 5-year DFS was 54%. The viability of the tumor after neoadjuvant chemotherapy plus or minus radiotherapy was measured according to the method of Salzer-Kuntschick et al [89] on surgical resection. In tumors with less than 10% viability on surgical resection, the 5-year DFS was 79%. In tumors with greater viability, the 5-year DFS was 31%.

The role of ifosfamide in Ewing's sarcoma family of tumors

In the early 1980s, treatment with ifosfamide, with or without etoposide, produced responses in patients who had soft tissue sarcomas who had relapsed after standard therapies [90–94]. This led to several protocols evaluating whether the replacement of cyclophosphamide with ifosfamide or the addition of ifosfamide would result in superior outcomes.

The Cooperative Ewing's Sarcoma Study-86 (CESS-86) performed between 1986 and 1991 stratified 301 patients who had localized ESB into standard-risk and high-risk cohorts based on tumor volume and location [30]. Patients who had tumor volumes greater than 100 mL, centrally-located tumors, or both were classified as high-risk. Patients in the standard-risk cohort were treated with VACA, whereas those in the high-risk cohort were treated with a combination of vincristine, actinomycin-D, ifosfamide, and doxorubicin (VAIA). The 5-year DFS was no different between cohorts (52% and 51%, respectively; $P = .92$), suggesting a clinical benefit to high-risk patients receiving intensified treatment incorporating ifosfamide.

The second national Ewing's Tumour Study (ET-2) performed in the United Kingdom between 1987 and 1993 evaluated 201 patients treated with VAIA [95]. The 5-year DFS was 62%, comparing favorably to the 5-year DFS of 36% documented in ET-1 where treatment consisted of VACA. The 5-year DFS found in ET-2 stratified by tumor location was 73% in patients who had extremity tumors, 55% in patients who had axial tumors, and 41% in patients who had pelvic tumors.

Several other small, nonrandomized trials reported improved survival with ifosfamide [31], whereas other studies performed in France and Italy found no effect [63,96]. The reasons for these contrasting results are not clear but may be partly caused by the fact that cyclophosphamide administered before 1986 was not given in what would now be accepted as maximally tolerated doses. Cyclophosphamide may be more effective if given at higher doses, but would then be associated with an increased risk for toxicity.

The addition of etoposide in the treatment of Ewing's sarcoma family of tumors

Preclinical and clinical studies have revealed a synergistic antitumor effect with the combined administration of etoposide and alkylators [91,97–99]. This synergistic effect is thought to occur from the inhibition of topoisomerase II by etoposide, thus increasing the cytotoxicity of alkylating agents such as ifosfamide by the impairment of the DNA uncoiling necessary for the repair of alkylating agent–induced DNA damage. In other studies, the effectiveness of etoposide and alkylators has also been found to improve with fractionated administration [100,101].

The small ES-87 study performed at SJCRH between 1987 and 1991 involved 26 patients and demonstrated that the combined administration of ifosfamide and etoposide (IE) in untreated patients who have EFT is very active [102]. Clinical responses were seen in 96% of patients.

A study performed at the Rizzoli Orthopaedic Institute between 1988 and 1991 involved 82 patients and evaluated the REN-2 protocol, a six-drug regimen that added IE to VACA in the maintenance setting. A 5-year EFS of 51% was noted. This outcome was not significantly different from that seen in a prior study using the REN-1 protocol of VACA without IE that revealed a 5-year DFS of 49% [82]. Although these results suggest no benefit from the addition of IE to VACA, the two new drugs were delivered only after local therapy in the REN-2 protocol. The REN-3 protocol, evaluated in 157 patients between 1991 and 1997, was developed to study the addition of ifosfamide in the neoadjuvant setting. The 5-year DFS was 71% in this study with an improved histologic response as measured by tumor viability when compared with tissue samples from the REN-1 and REN-2 protocols [74].

Two large randomized trials evaluated the impact of etoposide in the treatment of EFT. The first POG and Children's Cancer Group (POG-CCG) Ewing trial (POG-8850/CCG-7881) randomized patients to receive VACA plus or minus IE [33]. 398 patients who had localized disease were enrolled between 1988 and 1992. The addition of IE led to a significant improvement in outcome, with a 5-year DFS of 69% versus 54% ($P = .005$) in those who did not receive IE. The European Intergroup Cooperative Ewing's Sarcoma Study-92 (EICESS-92) performed between 1992 and 1999 stratified 470 patients into standard-risk and high-risk categories [103]. Patients were classified as high-risk if their tumor volume was greater than 200 mL. The standard-risk cohort was randomized to receive VACA or VAIA; the high-risk cohort was randomized to receive VAIA or etoposide, vincristine, actinomycin-D, ifosfamide, and doxorubicin (EVAIA). Standard-risk patients receiving VAIA had an improved 5-year DFS (79% versus 71%). High-risk patients receiving EVAIA also had an improved 5-year DFS (62% versus 54%) that was not statistically significant.

Trials of dose intensification

The incorporation of granulocyte colony-stimulating factor (G-CSF) into chemotherapeutic regimens has allowed for dose-intensification of multi-agent therapy by increasing the total dose per cycle [83,104,105] or by shortening the interval of time between treatments [106]. This approach in EFT is attractive because of the sensitivity of these tumors to alkylating agents [84–86,91], which have a steep dose-response curve. Additionally, by decreasing the interval between cycles, the recovery of partially resistant cells may be limited.

The EW-92 study performed at SJCRH between 1992 and 1996 evaluated the role of an aggressive dose-intensified induction phase regimen using vincristine, doxorubicin, and cyclophosphamide plus IE, followed by a prolonged maintenance phase with intensification of alkylating agents and etoposide [83]. In this study, 34 patients who had localized disease were randomized to receive vincristine, doxorubicin, and cyclophosphamide plus IE with either standard-dose cyclophosphamide or high-dose cyclophosphamide in the maintenance phase. Additionally, all patients received 1.4 (minimum increase for ifosfamide) to 3.0 (maximum increase for doxorubicin) times the dose prescribed during the earlier ES-87 study [102]. The estimated 3-year EFS was 60% with no significant difference between arms. Within the planned 8 weeks, 94% of patients completed the dose-intensified induction, but only 60% to 70% of patients were able to complete the maintenance therapy, and significant toxicities were noted, including an 8% incidence of treatment-related myeloid malignancies. With this schedule, hematologic toxicity was found to be dose-limiting and secondary myeloid malignancies were increased when results were compared with those of patients treated with more standard doses of chemotherapy [107–109].

Investigators at Memorial Sloan-Kettering Cancer Center (MSKCC) evaluated the use of a high-dose, short-term chemotherapy regimen between 1991 and 2001 in 68 patients who had a large tumor volume or disease metastatic to the bone or bone marrow. The P6 protocol used in this study consists of alternating courses of high-dose vincristine, doxorubicin, and cyclophosphamide (vincristine 2 mg/m^2, doxorubicin 75 mg/m^2, and cyclophosphamide 4200 mg/m^2), and IE (ifosfamide 1800 mg/m^2 and etoposide 100 mg/m^2) [110]. For the 44 patients who had locoregional disease, the 4-year EFS was 82%, which was not significantly better than results obtained with conventional therapy.

The second POG-CCG Ewing trial, (POG-9354/CCG-7942) performed from 1995 to 1998, randomized 492 patients to either 30 weeks or 48 weeks of alternating courses of vincristine, doxorubicin, and cyclophosphamide with IE. The 5-year EFS was 76% for the 30-week arm and 75% for the 48-week arm with no significant difference in outcome between the standard and the dose-intensified arms [111]. This prospective randomized trial demonstrated no increased risk for treatment-related acute myeloblastic leukemia (t-AML) with dose-intensive therapy (Smitha Bhatia, MD, personal communication, 2004).

Thus, for patients who have localized disease, dose intensification has not been a viable treatment option, particularly in light of the significant toxicities associated with these regimens. Questions remain, however, as to the best schedule for adjuvant chemotherapy.

Current standard of care

Current recommendations are for treatment with neoadjuvant chemotherapy followed by local control with surgical excision if the lesion is resectable. Surgery is particularly preferable in young children who may suffer from significant retardation of bone growth by radiotherapy, but may be complicated if prosthetic appliances must be placed. Radiation therapy should be employed for patients who do not have a surgical option that would preserve function and for those whose resections have been performed with inadequate margins. The IESS group recommends doses of 45 Gy to the original disease site with a 10.8-Gy boost for patients who have gross residual disease. For patients who have microscopic residual disease only, the recommendation is for 45 Gy with a 5.4-Gy boost. If there is no residual disease after surgical resection, no adjuvant radiotherapy is recommended.

Given the data of Grier et al [33] in the first POG-CCG study, the current standard chemotherapy for the treatment of EFT in the United States has evolved to include vincristine, doxorubicin, and cyclophosphamide with IE. Although dactinomycin is not routinely used in the United States, it is still included by some European groups with similar outcomes [74].

Treatment of metastatic disease

Approximately 20% to 25% of patients who have EFT have overt metastases at the time of diagnosis [24,27,112,113]. Patients who present with metastatic disease continue to have a poor prognosis with a 5-year relapse free survival

(RFS) rate of 30% [27]. There is a trend toward better survival for those with lung involvement alone as compared with those with bone metastases or a combination of lung and bone disease [114]. Many patients who have metastatic disease at diagnosis respond well to therapy used in patients who have localized disease. In most cases, however, the disease is only partially controlled or recurs despite treatment [113].

The IESS I and IESS II treated a total of 122 patients who had metastatic disease using VACA between 1975 and 1983 and found a 5-year DFS of 30% [115]. The ET-1 study treated 22 patients who had metastatic disease using VACA between 1978 and 1986 and found only a 9% 5-year DFS, paralleling their poorer outcome with localized disease when compared with the IESS data [69].

In the ET-2 study, which was performed between 1987 and 1993 and included 42 patients who had advanced disease, ifosfamide was added to the treatment regimen in the metastatic setting [23]. The 5-year DFS was 23% in these patients treated with VAIA, suggesting improved outcomes over those patients treated with VACA in the ET-1 study. However, there remains debate as to whether ifosfamide is superior to cyclophosphamide for patients who have metastatic Ewing sarcoma.

The first POG-CCG trial, performed between 1988 and 1992, randomized 120 patients who had metastatic disease to receive either VACA or VACA plus IE [114]. Unlike in the localized setting, no benefit was seen with the addition of IE for those who had metastatic disease (22% versus 22%, respectively, $P = .81$). EICESS evaluated 171 patients who had metastatic disease treated with EVAIA and found a 27% 5-year DFS [113]. When stratified by site of metastases, patients who had lung involvement only had a 34% 5-year DFS, patients who had bone or bone marrow involvement had a 28% 5-year DFS, and patients who had disease in the lungs and bones had a 14% 5-year DFS. Of the patients who had lung involvement, those treated with whole lung irradiation had a 40% 5-year DFS.

The efficacy of the high dose-intensity P6 protocol used at MSKCC was evaluated in six patients who had metastatic disease limited to the lungs and in 18 patients who had widespread metastatic disease [110]. The 4-year EFS was 12% in this population. Four patients (17%) died of treatment-related toxicities. The role of dose-intensification in the metastatic setting was also evaluated in the first POG-CCG trial, which included 60 patients placed on regimen C, a dose-intensified VACA plus IE regimen that was based on the P6 protocol [114]. The 5-year EFS was 26% with a high rate of significant toxicity including a 23% incidence of treatment-associated AML. The EW-92 study of dose-intensification performed at SJCRH included 19 patients who had metastatic disease [83]. The 5-year EFS was 27%, again showing no significant improvement in outcome with dose-intensification.

Current standard of care

The standard treatment of metastatic EFT includes chemotherapy combined with radiotherapy to all sites of gross disease, and possible selected surgical excision. This treatment often results in complete or partial responses; however, the overall cure rate remains approximately 20% [113,115,116].

The results from the first POG-CCG trial revealed no benefit from the addition of IE to a standard regimen of VACA [114]. These patients may thus be treated with vincristine, doxorubicin, and cyclophosphamide, reserving ifosfamide with etoposide for progression of disease on this regimen or in the situation of comprised cardiac function.

Radiation therapy to the primary tumor site and to sites of metastatic disease should be considered, but may be limited in an effort to preserve marrow function. Fractionated radiation therapy doses totaling between 45 Gy and 56 Gy should be used for metastatic disease of bone and soft tissue. At MSKCC, all patients who have pulmonary metastasis undergo WLI if complete resolution of disease has been achieved with chemotherapy alone [113,117,118]. The radiation dose for WLI is based on the amount of lung to be treated and pulmonary function, and typically consists of doses between 12 Gy and 15 Gy.

Treatment of progressive and relapsed disease

The outcome is poor once patients have relapsed, particularly for those relapsing within 2 years of diagnosis [27]. A recent study from SJCRH revealed a 17% 5-year postrecurrence survival. Those who had relapse more than 2 years after diagnosis, those who had local recurrence alone that could be treated with radical surgery and intensive chemotherapy, and those who had isolated pulmonary metastases treated with WLI fared better [119].

Studies performed in the early 1980s found significant responses in patients who had relapsed disease who were treated with ifosfamide with or without etoposide [90–94]. Of 72 patients treated with IE, 30 achieved a complete or partial response (combined data from two separate trials) [91,94].

Phase 1 and 2 studies of topotecan [120–123] and irinotecan [124,125] as single agents have shown modest activity in patients who have refractory disease. A phase 2 POG study evaluating the combination of cyclophosphamide and topotecan has resulted in responses in 36% of patients who have recurrent disease [126] and is considered a reasonable second-line option for patients progressing on vincristine, doxorubicin, and cyclophosphamide.

Based on these data, IE should be considered in patients who have not previously received these agents [91]. Other options include treatment with cyclophosphamide and topotecan or cisplatin and irinotecan.

Stem cell transplantation in the treatment of Ewing's sarcoma family of tumors

In an effort to improve outcome, particularly for high-risk patients, the role high-dose myeloablative therapy followed by stem cell rescue has been investigated. It was hoped that increased dose-intensity would increase the fraction of tumor cells destroyed, thus leading to an increased probability of long-term EFS. Several small series and case reports suggested improved clinical outcomes with stem cell transplantation (SCT) [113,127–139]; however, larger studies of SCT have been performed with conflicting data. The clinical findings of these trials are difficult to compare, as each study used variable eligibility criteria, induction protocols, myeloablative regimens, and sources of stem cells (autologous peripheral blood, autologous bone marrow, or allogeneic bone marrow).

The first study by the EICESS group evaluating the role of SCT in EFT involved 17 high-risk patients who had either multifocal disease (n=7) or recurrent disease (n=10) treated between 1986 and 1994 [140]. Eight of the 17 patients were alive and free of disease after consolidation therapy. These patients were previously treated with VACA, VAIA, or EVAIA and all had experienced at least a partial response before initiation of high-dose therapy. Cytoreduction was performed with varying doses of melphalan and etoposide plus or minus carboplatin, and all received total body irradiation (TBI). Transplantation was performed with autologous peripheral stem cells in nine cases, autologous bone marrow stem cells in four cases, and allogeneic stem cells in the remaining four cases. Some patients received additional treatment with IL-2 after reconstitution. The investigators compared the outcome of this cohort with the outcome of a matched cohort from a prior study for which the DFS was estimated to be zero. Although this estimation was likely overly pessimistic, the results of this study suggested that consolidation with high-dose therapy had provided benefit to a high-risk group of patients.

The National Cancer Institute (NCI) reported on 66 patients deemed high-risk based on having either metastatic disease or a primary tumor of the trunk, humerus, or femur who received consolidation with high-dose therapy followed by SCT [141]. Induction chemotherapy was based on one of three sequential clinical protocols offered at the NCI. Cytoreduction involved TBI followed by vincristine, doxorubicin, and cyclophosphamide. Notably, the radiotherapy dose was 8 Gy, a dose that is substantially lower than that used in many other trials. Additionally, the doses of chemotherapy used during cytoreduction were not significantly different from those used during induction. With this treatment regimen, no improvement in EFS was seen, suggesting no benefit for the role of SCT in EFT. When interpreting these data, the less stringent definition of high-risk disease and the less intensive dosing of the cytoreduction regimen used in this trial must be taken into account.

The CCG initiated a prospective trial of intensive induction chemotherapy followed by SCT consolidation for patients who had high-risk disease in an effort to resolve the conflicting results of the EICESS and NCI studies [142]. CCG-7951 was performed between 1996 and 1998 and enrolled 32 patients who had metastatic disease to the bone or bone marrow. These patients received the CCG-7881 protocol for induction and melphalan, etoposide, and TBI for consolidation, followed by autologous SCT. The first POG-CCG trial, in which patients were treated with a similar induction protocol but did not receive SCT, reported a 17% EFS in patients who had metastatic disease to the bone or bone marrow [143], thus providing a measure for comparison. The 2-year EFS in this CCG trial was 16%, revealing no advantage for high-dose therapy. Of note, eight of the 32 patients were not able to receive the high-dose therapy because of incomplete response, progressive disease, or death caused by treatment-related toxicity.

This lack of benefit from SCT was again seen in a study performed at MSKCC between 1990 and 1998 that evaluated 21 patients who had newly diagnosed EFT with metastasis to the bone or bone marrow [144]. All patients received induction with the P6 protocol. Those patients who had a complete response (CR) or very good partial response (VGPR) went on to consolidation with either melphalan and TBI or thiotepa and carboplatin. After induction, 90% of patients achieved a CR or VGPR. Ten, however, had progressive disease while receiving chemotherapy or shortly after chemotherapy, and were not eligible for SCT. Eight patients went on to consolidation with melphalan and TBI. Of these, one patient maintained a CR at more than 7 years, four had relapsed disease, two died from toxicity, and one died of an unrelated cause. Three patients received thiotepa and carboplatin for consolidation. All three relapsed within 3 to 4 months after treatment. The reported 3-year EFS was 5%.

The experiences at the NCI, CCG, and MSKCC, each of which involved unselected patients treated with SCT, revealed no benefit from the inclusion of myeloablative therapy in the treatment of EFT. The positive results noted in the EICESS study may be attributable to the fact that all patients enrolled in that study had already achieved a partial or complete remission at the start of the trial. Thus, a selection bias toward those who had more responsive disease may have affected their results.

Still under study is the role of allogeneic bone marrow transplantation, as is discussed later.

Consolidation regimens and their relation to outcome

The effect of various consolidation regimens on outcome has been evaluated in various case series and retrospective reports but has not been studied in a prospective randomized trial. One small series evaluated 11 patients who had metastatic or recurrent high-risk disease who received consolidation with thiotepa, melphalan, and busulfan and found a 62% 3-year DFS [145]. The usefulness of conditioning regimens involving this triple alkylating agent regimen may warrant future study.

A report from the European Bone Marrow Transplant Registry (EBMTR) evaluated 63 patients who had EFT who were treated with SCT between 1982 and 1992 [146]. The consolidation regimens used varied significantly and included combinations of melphalan, carmustine, etoposide, busulfan, and TBI. Patients treated with TBI had inferior outcomes in this study. Superior results were noted in those treated with a combination of melphalan and busulfan.

A second report by the EBMTR evaluated 111 patients treated with SCT between 1978 and 1997 [147] and evaluated outcome based on whether or not busulfan was included in the consolidation regimen. The 5-year overall survival (OS) for patients who received busulfan was 44% versus 23% in those who did not ($P = .061$). In the subset of patients who had pulmonary involvement, the OS was 66% for those who received busulfan versus 39% in those who did not. In those who had localized high-risk disease, the OS was 75% for those who received busulfan versus 38% in those who did not.

Because these data are drawn from a registry, the EBMTR findings reflect only the application of SCT to those patients who have already achieved a remission with conventional therapy. Thus, these results do not apply to all patients at initial diagnosis. Nevertheless, the possibility that high-dose regimens including busulfan can improve the prognosis for high-risk EFT is an important one and is being tested in a randomized prospective trial by the European cooperative group for the study of EFT (EURO-E.W.I.N.G. 99).

Allogeneic stem cell transplantation

There seems to be good biologic rationale for recurrence of Ewing sarcoma following autologous SCT. Several investigators have found that EFT cells are detectable by PCR in stem cell grafts, even after positive selection for CD34+ cells [142,148]. This minimal residual disease may contribute to disease recurrence after autologous SCT. Preclinical studies using ex vivo purging by electroporation of antisense oligonucleotides seem to be promising and may improve outcome after autologous transplantation in the future [149]. Evaluation of a monoclonal antibody for the purpose of immunologic purging of residual disease is ongoing [150]. Although the eradication of all disease from the harvested stem cells may lead to improved outcome with autologous SCT, it is unclear if or when this will be clinically feasible.

The role of allogeneic SCT has been of interest because of the possibility for contaminated stem cells in the autologous setting and the potential for a clinically significant graft-versus-tumor (GVT) effect. The expression of surface proteins derived from the characteristic gene fusion product seen in EFT suggests the potential for a GVT phenomenon [151–153]. Additionally, models of EFT immunotherapy have implicated natural killer cells, suggesting down-regulation of major histocompatibility complex class I molecules in EFT in vivo [154].

The consensus of two workshops on high-risk EFT was that allogeneic SCT conferred no benefit when compared with autologous SCT and is associated with a higher complication rate [140,155]. This consensus, however, is based on limited evidence. Studies evaluating the utility of allogeneic SCT have involved low numbers of patients and have reported contradictory results [140,156]. In these experiences, patients were typically selected for allogeneic transplant only if postconsolidation marrow studies revealed persistent tumor cells, possibly causing a selection bias for treatment-refractory patients.

An Australian study performed between 1984 and 1996 reported on 18 patients who had metastatic EFT (the sites of metastases were not specified in the study) who were previously treated with VACA and then underwent SCT

[156]. Melphalan and etoposide were used for cytoreduction. The 4-year OS was 26%. Of note, six of the 18 patients underwent allogeneic transplantation, three of whom were rendered relapse-free. In two other studies, three of four patients who received allogeneic SCT were relapse-free at 6, 29, and 51 months after transplantation [131,157].

Current recommendations

The role of SCT in this disease remains under evaluation. Because high-dose chemotherapy with or without total-body irradiation followed by stem cell support has not shown improvement in EFS for patients who have advanced EFT, the use of SCT in the treatment of EFT should only be performed as part of a prospective investigational trial.

Risk for secondary malignancy after curative therapy

Treatment-related acute myeloblastic leukemia and myelodysplastic syndrome (t-AML/MDS) have been reported in 1% to 2% of survivors of EFT [158–160]. These secondary malignancies occur most commonly between 2 and 5 years following diagnosis [159,160]. The advent of protocols that include intensification of alkylators and topoisomerase-II inhibitors has resulted in a significant increase in the incidence of t-AML/MDS [144]. The cumulative incidence of t-AML/MDS was 8% in survivors of the MSKCC P6 protocol [161] and 22.7% at 4 years for patients treated on the POG-8850/CCG-7881 regimen C, a rate significantly higher than that seen in patients treated less intensively on the same protocol with regimens A and B [109]. At SJCRH, patients treated on the EW92 protocol had a cumulative incidence of t-AML/MDS of 8% compared with 0% treated on the ES87 protocol in which the same drugs were used but at lower doses [162].

Although these nonrandomized trials suggest an increased risk for t-AML/MDS with intensified treatment regimens, the second POG-CCG Ewing trial, which was a prospective randomized trial, revealed no increased risk for t-AML/MDS with intensified treatment (Smitha Bhatia, MD, personal communication, 2004).

Survivors of EFT additionally appear to remain at increased risk for developing a second solid tumor throughout their lifetime with a cumulative risk of 5% to 10% at 15 to 20 years from diagnosis [108,158,163]. The risk for developing solid tumors seems to be greatest in patients treated with radiation therapy, and secondary sarcomas usually develop within the prior radiation field [108,160,164]. In one multi-institutional study that included 266 survivors of EFT, the cumulative incidence of a secondary sarcoma was 6.5% [108]. The risk for developing a sarcoma following radiation therapy is dose-dependent, with higher doses of radiation associated with an increased risk for sarcoma development. One retrospective study reported that patients who received 60 Gy or more had a 20% incidence of a second malignancy. For those who received between 48 Gy and 60 Gy, the incidence was 5%. For those who received less than 48 Gy, there was no increased risk for a second malignancy [108].

Current clinical trials and prospects for future studies

The prognosis for patients who have EFT has improved dramatically with the advent of combined modality therapy [62–65]. Despite these advancements in therapy, a significant proportion of patients develop recurrent disease and eventually succumb to their disease. Therefore, continued investigation of novel treatment strategies is important to further improve the outcome of these patients.

Immunohistochemical studies performed on EFT have shown that approximately 70% of samples express c-kit, with strong and diffuse staining seen in 30% of cases [165]. The activation of c-kit in EFT seems to be involved in cell survival [166]. Although the usefulness of the tyrosine kinase inhibitor STI-571 (imatinib) in the treatment of chronic myeloid leukemia [167], Philadelphia chromosome–positive acute lymphoid leukemia [168], and gastrointestinal stromal tumors [169] has been found to be significant, its use in EFT has not been shown to be effective [170].

The Children's Oncology Group is currently conducting a phase 3 randomized study of interval-compressed versus standard chemotherapy in patients who have newly diagnosed, localized EFT. This multicenter trial will randomize patients to receive dose-intensive chemotherapy on either a 14-day or a 21-day schedule to determine whether increasing the dose intensity of all drugs simultaneously, through a reduction of the interval between chemotherapy cycles or interval compression, improves survival. Filgrastim will be used for hematologic support. Data supporting this experimental interval compression come from a nonrandomized pilot study that used hematopoietic growth factors to allow for interval-dose compression. The interval between courses of chemotherapy was decreased from 21 days to 14 days in this study [106]. Approximately 528 patients will be accrued for this study within 4 to 5 years.

The European Ewing Tumour Working Initiative of National Groups Ewing Tumour Studies 1999 (EURO-EWING-INTERGROUP-EE99) is a phase 3 randomized study of standard induction therapy followed by consolidation therapy with vincristine, actinomycin D, and ifosfamide (VAI) versus VAC versus busulfan, melphalan, and autologous SCT, with or without radiotherapy or surgery, in patients who have EFT. This study hopes to accrue approximately 1200 patients within 7 years. Treatment is stratified according to tumor volume, histologic response, and metastasis. Low-risk patients will be randomized to receive either VAI or VAC for consolidation chemotherapy. Nonmetastatic high-risk patients will be randomized to receive either VAI consolidation chemotherapy or busulfan and melphalan followed by autologous stem cell transplant. Patients who have pulmonary metastasis at diagnosis will be randomized to receive either VAI consolidation chemotherapy and WLI or busulfan and melphalan followed by autologous SCT.

Recent work on insulin-like growth factor (IGF) receptors has shown that these receptors play an essential role in the pathogenesis of EFT. The insulin-like growth factor-I pathway (IGF-1/IGF-1R) is actively involved in the cell transformation and inhibition of apoptosis induced by EWS-FLI1 [171,172]. Thus, it is possible that the inhibition of the IGF-1R or downstream components of the pathway such as PI3-K or Akt may lead to antitumor activity or potentiation of standard chemotherapeutic agents [172,173]. In a trial using IGF-1 receptor antisense oligonucleotides in nude mice, it was demonstrated that survival was increased and that tumor formation was delayed compared with untreated mice. Additionally, it was shown that inhibition of the IGF-1 receptors enhanced the sensitivity of tumor cells to doxorubicin [174]. Thus, IGF-1 receptor antisense oligonucleotides may have a future role in treating patients who have EFT by reducing the malignant potential of the sarcoma and by augmenting conventional chemotherapeutic agents. Additionally, the inhibition of downstream elements of PI3-K,such as mTOR, may lead to antitumor activity and thus rapamycin and its derivatives may prove useful in the treatment of EFT [175].

The next few years will mark an important time for the treatment of EFT with the development of numerous targeted agents, some of which will have an impact on this family of sarcomas.

References

[1] Ewing J. Diffuse endothelioma of bone. Proc NY Pathol Soc 1921:17–24.

[2] Delattre O, Zucman J, Melot T, et al. The Ewing family of tumors: a subgroup of small-round-cell tumors defined by specific chimeric transcripts. N Engl J Med 1994;331:294–9.

[3] Schmidt D, Herrman C, Jurgens J, et al. Malignant peripheral neuroectodermal tumor and its necessary distinction from Ewing's sarcoma. Cancer 1991;68:2251–9.

[4] Parham DM, Hijazi Y, Steinberg SM, et al. Neuroectodermal differentiation in Ewing's sarcoma family of tumors does not predict tumor behavior. Hum Pathol 1999;30(8):911–8.

[5] Luksch R, Sampietro G, Collini P, et al. Prognostic value of clinicopathologic characteristics including neuroectodermal differentiation in osseous Ewing's sarcoma family of tumors in children. Tumori 1999;85(2):101–7.

[6] Bacci G, Ferrari S, Bertoni F, et al. Neoadjuvant chemotherapy for peripheral malignant neuroectodermal tumor of bone: recent experience at the Istituto Rizzoli. J Clin Oncol 2000; 18:885–92.

[7] Wexler LH, Meyer WH, Parham DM, et al. Neural differentiation and prognosis in peripheral primitive neuroectodermal tumor. J Clin Oncol 2000;18:2187–8.

[8] Ries LAG, Eisner MP, Kosary CL, et al. SEER Cancer Statistics Review, 1975–2001. Bethesda (MD): National Cancer Institute; 2004.

[9] Buckley JD, Pendergrass TW, Buckley CM, et al. Epidemiology of osteosarcoma and Ewing's sarcoma in childhood: a study of 305 cases from the Children's Cancer Group. Cancer 1998; 83:1440–8.

[10] Gurney JG, Severson RK, Davis S, et al. Incidence of cancer in children in the United States. Cancer 1995;75:2186–95.

[11] Polednak AP. Primary bone cancer incidence in black and white residents of New York state. Cancer 1985;55:2883–8.

[12] Glass A, Fraumeni J. Epidemiology of bone cancer in children. J Natl Cancer Inst 1970;44: 187–99.
[13] Li F, Tu J, Liu F, et al. Rarity of Ewing's sarcoma in China. Lancet 1980;1:1255.
[14] Gou W, Xu W, Huvos AG, et al. Comparative frequency of bone sarcomas among different racial groups. Chin Med J (Engl) 1999;112:1101–4.
[15] Zucman-Rossi J, Batzer MA, Stoneking M, et al. Interethnic polymorphism of EWS intron 6: genome plasticity mediated by Alu retroposition and recombination. Hum Genet 1997;99: 357–63.
[16] Fraumeni J. Stature and malignant tumors of bone in childhood and adolescence. Cancer 1967;20:967–73.
[17] Pendergrass TW, Foulkes MA, Robison LL, et al. Stature and Ewing's sarcoma in childhood. Am J Pediatr Hematol Oncol 1984;6:33–9.
[18] Winn DM, Li FP, Robison LL, et al. A case-control study of the etiology of Ewing's sarcoma. Cancer Epidemiol Biomarkers Prev 1992;1:525–32.
[19] Holly EA, Aston DA, Ahn DK, et al. Ewing's bone sarcoma, paternal occupational exposure, and other factors. Am J Epidemiol 1992;135:135.
[20] Hartley AL, Birch JM, Blair CV, et al. Cancer Incidence in the families of children with Ewing's sarcoma. J Natl Cancer Inst 1991;83(13):955–6.
[21] Novakovic B, Tucker MA, Wexler L, et al. Risk of cancer in families of patients with Ewing's sarcoma family of tumors. Ann Meet Am Assoc Cancer Res 1994;35:A1729.
[22] Li FP, Fraumeni JF, Mulvihill JJ, et al. A cancer family syndrome in twenty-four kindreds. Cancer Res 1988;48:5358–62.
[23] Craft A, Cotterill S, Malcolm A, et al. Ifosfamide-containing chemotherapy in Ewing's sarcoma: The Second United Kingdom Children's Cancer Study Group and The Medical Research Council Ewing's Tumor Study. J Clin Oncol 1998;16(11):3628–33.
[24] Donaldson SS, Torrey M, Link MP, et al. A multidisciplinary study investigating radiotherapy in Ewing's sarcoma: end results of POG #8346. Int J Radiat Oncol Biol Phys 1998; 42(1):125–35.
[25] Kennedy JG, Eustace S, Caufield R, et al. Extraskeletal Ewing's sarcoma: a case report and review of the literature. Spine 2000;25:1996–9.
[26] Coffin CM, Dehner LP. Neurogenic tumors of soft tissue. In: Coffin CM, Dehner LP, O'Shea PA, editors. Pediatric soft tissue tumors: a clinical, pathological, and therapeutic approach. Baltimore (MD): Williams and Wilkins; 1997. p. 80–132.
[27] Cotterill SJ, Ahrens S, Paulussen M, et al. Prognostic factors in Ewing's tumor of bone: analysis of 975 patients from the European Intergroup Cooperative Ewing's Sarcoma Study Group. J Clin Oncol 2000;18(17):3108–14.
[28] Bacci G, Ferrari S, Longhi A, et al. Prognostic significance of serum LDH in Ewing's sarcoma of bone. Oncol Rep 1999;6(4):807–11.
[29] Bacci G, Picci P, Mercuri M, et al. Predictive factors of histological response to primary chemotherapy in Ewing's sarcoma. Acta Oncol 1998;37(7–8):671–6.
[30] Paulussen M, Ahrens S, Dunst J, et al. Localized Ewing tumor of bone: final results of the cooperative Ewing's Sarcoma Study CESS 86. J Clin Oncol 2001;19(6):1818–29.
[31] Rosito P, Mancini AF, Rondelli R, et al. Italian Cooperative Study for the treatment of children and young adults with localized Ewing sarcoma of bone: a preliminary report of 6 years of experience. Cancer 1999;86(3):421–8.
[32] Shankar AG, Pinkerton CR, Atra A. Local therapy and other factors influencing site of relapse in patients with localised Ewing's sarcoma. United Kingdom Children's Cancer Study Group (UKCCSG). Eur J Cancer 1999;35(12):1698–704.
[33] Grier HE, Krailo MD, Tarbell NJ, et al. Addition of ifosfamide and etoposide to standard chemotherapy for Ewing's sarcoma and primitive neuroectodermal tumor of bone. N Engl J Med 2003;348(8):694–701.
[34] Aurias A, Rimbaud C, Buffe D, et al. Chromosomal translocations in Ewing's sarcoma. N Engl J Med 1983;309:496–7.

[35] Turc-Carel C, Philip I, Berger M-P, et al. Chromosomal translocations in Ewing's sarcoma. N Engl J Med 1983;309:497.

[36] Turc-Carel C, Aurias A, Mugneret F, et al. Chromosomes in Ewing's sarcoma. I. An evaluation of 85 cases and remarkable consistency of t(11;22)(q24;q12). Cancer Genet Cytogenet 1988; 32:229.

[37] Denny CT. Gene rearrangements in Ewing's sarcoma. Cancer Invest 1996;14(1):83–8.

[38] Bridge J. Cytogenetic and molecular cytogenetic techniques in orthopaedic surgery. J Bone Joint Surg Am 1993;75(4):606.

[39] Zucman J, Delattre O, Desmaze C, et al. Cloning and characterization of the Ewing's sarcoma and peripheral neuroepithelioma t(11;22) translocation breakpoint. Genes Chromosomes Cancer 1992;5:271.

[40] De Alava E, Kawai A, Healey JH, et al. EWS-FLI1 fusion transcript structure is an independent determinant of prognosis in Ewing's sarcoma. J Clin Oncol 1998;16(4):1248–55.

[41] De Avala E, Panizo A, Antonescu CR, et al. Association of EWS-FLI1 type 1 fusion with lower proliferative rate in Ewing's sarcoma. Am J Pathol 2000;156:849–55.

[42] Peter M, Couturier J, Pacquement H, et al. A new member of the ETS family fused to EWS in Ewing tumors. Oncogene 1997;14:1159.

[43] Urano F, Umezawa A, Yabe H, et al. Molecular analysis of Ewing's sarcoma: another fusion gene, EWS-E1AF, available for diagnosis. Jpn J Cancer Res 1998;89(7):703–11.

[44] Ozaki T, Paulussen M, Poremba C, et al. Genetic imbalances revealed by comparative genomic hybridization in Ewing tumors. Genes Chromosomes Cancer 2001;32(2):164–71.

[45] Huang HY, Illei PB, Zhao Z, et al. Ewing sarcomas with p53 mutation or p16/p14 ARF homozygous deletion: a highly lethal subset associated with poor chemoresponse. J Clin Oncol 2005;23(3):548–58.

[46] Amir G, Issakov J, Meller I, et al. Expression of p53 gene product and cell proliferation marker Ki-67 in Ewing's sarcoma: correlation with clinical outcome. Hum Pathol 2002;33: 170–4.

[47] Wei G, Antonescu CR, de Alava E, et al. Prognostic impact on INK4 deletion in Ewing's sarcoma. Cancer 2000;89:793–9.

[48] Hattinger CM, Rumpler S, Strehl S, et al. Prognostic impact of deletions at 1p36 and numerical aberrations in Ewing tumors. Genes Chromosomes Cancer 1999;24(3):243–54.

[49] Dahlin DC, Coventry MB, Scanlon P. Ewing's sarcoma. J Bone Joint Surg Am 1961;43A: 185–92.

[50] Bhansali SK, Desai PB. Ewing's sarcoma: observation on 107 cases. J Bone Joint Surg Am 1963;45A:541–53.

[51] Phelan JT, Cabrera A. Ewing's sarcoma. Surg Gynecol Obstet 1964;118:795–800.

[52] Falk S, Alpert M. Five-year survival of patients with Ewing's sarcoma. Surg Gynecol Obstet 1967;124:319–24.

[53] Freeman AI, Sachatello C, Gaeta J, et al. An analysis of Ewing's tumor in children at Roswell Park Memorial Institute. Cancer 1972;29:1563–9.

[54] Nesbit ME. Ewing's sarcoma. CA Cancer J Clin 1976;26:174–80.

[55] West DC, Grier HE, Swallow MM, et al. Detection of circulating tumor cells in patients with Ewing's sarcoma and peripheral primitive neuroectodermal tumor. J Clin Oncol 1997;15: 583–8.

[56] Zoubek A, Ladenstein R, Windhager R, et al. Predictive potential of testing for bone marrow involvement in Ewing tumor patients by RT-PCR: a preliminary evaluation. Int J Cancer 1998; 79:56–60.

[57] Fagnou C, Michon J, Peter M, et al. Presence of tumor cells in bone marrow but not in blood is associated with adverse prognosis in patients with Ewing's tumor. J Clin Oncol 1998;16: 1707–11.

[58] Schleiermacher G, Peter M, Oberlin O, et al. Increased risk of systemic relapses associated with bone marrow micrometastases and circulating tumor cells in localized Ewing tumor. J Clin Oncol 2003;21(1):85–91.

[59] Nesbit Jr ME, Gehan EA, Burgert Jr EO, et al. Multimodal therapy for the management of primary, nonmetastatic Ewing's sarcoma of bone: a long-term follow-up of the first intergroup study. J Clin Oncol 1990;8(10):1664–74.

[60] Jaffe N, Paed D, Traggis D, et al. Improved outlook for Ewing's sarcoma with combination chemotherapy (vincristine, actinomycin D and cyclophosphamide) and radiation therapy. Cancer 1976;38:1925–30.

[61] Rosen G, Caparros B, Mosende C, et al. Curability of Ewing's sarcoma and considerations for future therapeutic trials. Cancer 1978;41:888–99.

[62] Jurgens H, Exner U, Gadner H, et al. Multidisciplinary treatment of primary Ewing's sarcoma of bone: a 6-year experience of a European cooperative trial. Cancer 1988;61:23–32.

[63] Bacci G, Toni A, Avella M, et al. Long-term results in 144 localized Ewing's sarcoma patients treated with combined therapy. Cancer 1989;63:1477–86.

[64] Barbieri E, Emiliani E, Zini G, et al. Combined therapy of localized Ewing's sarcoma of bone: analysis of results in 100 patients. Int J Radiat Oncol Biol Phys 1990;19:1165–70.

[65] Kinsella TJ, Miser JS, Waller B, et al. Long-term follow-up of Ewing's sarcoma of bone treated with combined modality therapy. Int J Radiat Biol Phys 1991;20:389–95.

[66] Wunder JS, Paulian G, Huvos AG, et al. The histological response to chemotherapy as a predictor of the oncological outcome of operative treatment of Ewing sarcoma. J Bone Joint Surg Am 1998;80(7):1020–33.

[67] Oberlin O, Deley MC, Bui BN, et al. Prognostic factors in localized Ewing's tumours and peripheral neuroectodermal tumours: the third study of the French Society of Paediatric Oncology (EW88 study). Br J Cancer 2001;85(11):1646–54.

[68] Dyke JP, Panicek DM, Healey JH, et al. Osteogenic and Ewing sarcomas: estimation of necrotic fraction during induction chemotherapy with dynamic contrast-enhanced MR imaging. Radiology 2003;228(1):271–8.

[69] Craft AW, Cotterill SJ, Bullimore JA, et al. Long-term results from the first UKCCSG Ewing's tumor study (ET-1). Eur J Cancer 1997;33:1061–9.

[70] Ozaki T, Hillman A, Hoffman C, et al. Significance of surgical margin on the prognosis of patients with Ewing's sarcoma. Cancer 1996;78:892–900.

[71] Sluga M, Windhager R, Lang S, et al. The role of surgery and resection margins in the treatment of Ewing sarcoma. Clin Orthop 2001;392:394–9.

[72] Terek RM, Brien EW, Marcove RC, et al. Treatment of femoral Ewing's sarcoma. Cancer 1996;78:70–8.

[73] Ozaki T, Hillmann A, Hoffmann C, et al. Ewing's sarcoma of the femur. Acta Orthop Scand 1997;68:20–4.

[74] Bacci G, Mercuri M, Longhi A, et al. Neoadjuvant chemotherapy for Ewing's tumor of bone: recent experience at the Rizzoli Orthopaedic Institute. Eur J Cancer 2002;38:2243–51.

[75] Burgert EO, Nesbit ME, Garsney LA, et al. Multimodal therapy for the management of nonpelvic, localized Ewing's sarcoma of bone: Intergroup Study IESS-II. J Clin Oncol 1990; 8:1514–24.

[76] Dunst J, Hoffmann C, Ahrens S, et al. Surgery versus radiotherapy in Ewing's sarcoma with good prognosis. Analysis of the CESS 86 data. Strahlenther Onkol 1996;172:244–8.

[77] Wilkins RM, Pritchard DJ, Burgert EO, et al. Ewing's sarcoma of bone: Experience with 140 patients. Cancer 1986;58:2551–5.

[78] Merchant TE, Kushner BH, Sheldon JM, et al. Effect of low-dose radiation therapy when combined with surgical resection for Ewing sarcoma. Med Pediatr Oncol 1999;33:65–70.

[79] Bacci G, Ferrari S, Bertoni F, et al. Prognostic factors in non-metastatic Ewing's sarcoma of bone treated with adjuvant chemotherapy: Analysis of 359 patients at the Istituto Ostopedico Rizzoli. J Clin Oncol 2000;18:4–11.

[80] Schuck A, Rube C, Konemann S, et al. Postoperative radiotherapy in the treatment of Ewing tumors: influence of the interval between surgery and radiotherapy. Strahlenther Onkol 2002; 178:25–31.

[81] Dunst J, Jurgens H, Sauer R, et al. Radiation therapy in Ewing's sarcoma: an update of the CESS 86 trial. Int J Radiat Oncol Biol Phys 1995;32:919–30.

[82] Bacci G, Picci P, Ferrari S, et al. Neoadjuvant chemotherapy for Ewing's sarcoma of bone: no benefit observed after adding ifosfamide and etoposide to vincristine, actinomycin, cyclophosphamide, and doxorubicin in the maintenance phase - results of two sequential studies. Cancer 1998;82:1174–83.
[83] Marina NM, Pappo AS, Parham DM, et al. Chemotherapy dose-intensification for pediatric patients with Ewing's family of tumors and desmoplastic small round cell tumor: a feasibility study at St. Jude Children's Research Hospital. J Clin Oncol 1999;17:180–90.
[84] Haggard ME. Cyclophosphamide (NSC-26271) in the treatment of children with malignant neoplasms. Cancer Chemother Rep 1967;51:403–5.
[85] Samuels ML, Howe CD. Cyclophosphamide in the management of Ewing's sarcoma. Cancer 1967;20:961–6.
[86] Johnson R, Humphreys DR. Past failures and future possibilities in Ewing's sarcoma: experimental and preliminary clinical results. Cancer 1969;23:161–6.
[87] Oldham RK, Pomeroy TC. Treatment of Ewing's sarcoma with Adriamycin (NSC 123127). Cancer Chemother Rep 1972;56:635–9.
[88] Hayes FA, Thompson EI, Meyer WH, et al. Therapy for localized Ewing's sarcoma of bone. J Clin Oncol 1989;7:208–13.
[89] Salzer-Kuntschik M, Delling G, Beron G, et al. Morphological grades of regression in osteosarcoma after polychemotherapy–study COSS 80. J Cancer Res Clin Oncol 1983;106(Suppl): 21–4.
[90] Magrath I, Sandlund J, Raynor A, et al. A phase II study of ifosfamide in the treatment of recurrent sarcomas in young people. Cancer Chemother Pharmacol 1986;18(S2):S25–8.
[91] Miser JS, Kinsella TJ, Triche TJ, et al. Ifosfamide with mesna uroprotection and etoposide: an effective regimen in the treatment of recurrent sarcomas and other tumors of children and young adults. J Clin Oncol 1987;5:1191–8.
[92] Antman K, Ryan L, Elias A, et al. Response to ifosfamide and mesna: 124 previously treated patients with metastatic or unresectable sarcoma. J Clin Oncol 1989;7:126–31.
[93] Jurgens H, Exner U, Kuhl J, et al. High-dose ifosfamide with mesna uroprotection in Ewing's sarcoma. Cancer Chemother Pharmacol 1989;24(S1):S40–4.
[94] Kung FH, Pratt CB, Vega RA, et al. Ifosfamide/etoposide combination in the treatment of recurrent malignant solid tumors of childhood: a Pediatric Oncology Group Phase II study. Cancer 1993;71:1898–903.
[95] Craft ACS, Malcolm A, et al. Ifosfamide-containing chemotherapy in Ewing's sarcoma: The Second United Kingdom Children's Cancer Study Group and The Medical Research Council Ewing's Tumor Study. J Clin Oncol 1998;16:3628–33.
[96] Oberlin O, Habrand JL, Zucker JM, et al. No benefit of ifosfamide in Ewing's sarcoma: a nonrandomized study of the French Society of Pediatric Oncology. J Clin Oncol 1992;10: 1737–42.
[97] Lilly ER, Rosenberg MC, Elion GB, et al. Synergistic interactions between cyclophosphamide or melphalan and VP-16 in a human rhabdomyosarcoma xenograft. Cancer Res 1990;50: 284–7.
[98] Kung FH, Pratt CB, Vega RA, et al. Ifosfamide/etoposide combination in the treatment of recurrent malignant solid tumors of childhood. Cancer 1993;71:1898–903.
[99] Yazawa Y, Takagi T, Asakura S, et al. Effects of 4-hydroperoxyifosfamide in combination with other anticancer agents on human cancer cell lines. J Orthop Sci 1999;4:231–7.
[100] Kurowski V, Wagner T. Comparative pharmacokinetics of ifosfamide, 4-hydroxyifosfamide, chloroacetylaldehyde, and 2- and 3-dechloroethylifosfamide in patients on fractionated intravenous ifosfamide therapy. Cancer Chemother Pharmacol 1993;33:36–42.
[101] Clark PI, Slevin ML, Joel SP, et al. A randomized trial of two etoposide schedules in small-cell lung cancer: The influence of pharmacokinetics on efficacy and toxicity. J Clin Oncol 1994; 12:1427–35.
[102] Meyer WH, Kun L, Marina N, et al. Ifosfamide plus etoposide in newly diagnosed Ewing's sarcoma of bone. J Clin Oncol 1992;10:385–93.
[103] Paulussen M, Ahrens S, Braun-Munzinger G, et al. [EICESS 92 (European Intergroup Coop-

erative Ewing's Sarcoma Study)–preliminary results]. Klin Padiatr 1999;211(4):276–83 [in German].

[104] Kushner B, Meyers P, Gerald W, et al. Very-high-dose short-term chemotherapy for poor-risk peripheral primitive neuroectodermal tumors, including Ewing's sarcoma, in children and young adults. J Clin Oncol 1995;13:2796–804.

[105] Kushner BH, LaQuaglia MP, Wollner N, et al. Desmoplastic small-round cell tumor: Prolonged progression free survival with aggressive multi-modality therapy. J Clin Oncol 1996; 14:1526–31.

[106] Womer RB, Daller RT, Fenton JG, et al. Granulocyte colony stimulating factor permits dose intensification by interval compression in the treatment of Ewing's sarcomas and soft tissue sarcomas in children. Eur J Cancer 2000;36(1):87–94.

[107] Ruymann FB, Vietti T, Gehan E, et al. Cyclophosphamide dose escalation in combination with vincristine and actinomycin-D (VAC) in gross residual sarcoma: a pilot study without hematopoietic growth factor support evaluating toxicity and response. J Pediatr Hematol Oncol 1995;17:331–7.

[108] Kuttesch JF, Wexler LH, Marcus RB, et al. Second malignancies after Ewing's sarcoma: radiation dose-dependency of secondary sarcomas. J Clin Oncol 1996;14:2818–25.

[109] Miser J, Krailo M, Smith M, et al. Secondary leukemia (SL) or myelodysplastic syndrome (MDS) following therapy for Ewing's sarcoma (ES) [abstract]. Proc Am Soc Clin Oncol 1997; 16:518.

[110] Kolb EA, Kushner BH, Gorlick R, et al. Long-term event-free survival after intensive chemotherapy for Ewing's family of tumors in children and young adults. J Clin Oncol 2003;21(18): 3423–30.

[111] Granowetter L, Womer R, Devidas M, et al. Comparison of dose intensified and standard dose chemotherapy for the treatment of non-metastatic Ewing's sarcoma (ES) and primitive neuroectodermal tumor (PNET) of bone and soft tissue: a Pediatric Oncology Group-Children's Cancer Group phase III trial [abstract]. Med Pedriatr Oncol 2001;37:172.

[112] Raney RB, Asmar L, Newton Jr WA, et al. Ewing's sarcoma of soft tissues in childhood: a report from the Intergroup Rhabdomyosarcoma Study, 1972 to 1991. J Clin Oncol 1997; 15(2):574–82.

[113] Paulussen M, Ahrens S, Burdach S, et al. Primary metastatic (stage IV) Ewing tumor: survival analysis of 171 patients from the EICESS studies. European Intergroup Cooperative Ewing Sarcoma Studies. Ann Oncol 1998;9(3):275–81.

[114] Miser JS, Krailo MD, Tarbell NJ, et al. Treatment of metastatic Ewing's sarcoma or primitive neuroectodermal tumor of bone: evaluation of combination ifosfamide and etoposide–a Children's Cancer Group and Pediatric Oncology Group study. J Clin Oncol 2004;22(14): 2873–6.

[115] Cangir A, Vietti TJ, Gehan EA, et al. Ewing's sarcoma metastatic at diagnosis. Results and comparisons of two Intergroup Ewing's Sarcoma Studies. Cancer 1990;66(5):887–93.

[116] Pinkerton CR, Bataillard A, Guillo S, et al. Treatment strategies for metastatic Ewing's sarcoma. Eur J Cancer 2001;37(11):1338–44.

[117] Madero L, Muñoz A, Sánchez de Toledo J, et al. Megatherapy in children with high-risk Ewing's sarcoma in first complete remission. Bone Marrow Transplant 1998;21(8):795–9.

[118] Spunt SL, McCarville MB, Kun LE, et al. Selective use of whole-lung irradiation for patients with Ewing sarcoma family tumors and pulmonary metastases at the time of diagnosis. J Pediatr Hematol Oncol 2001;23(2):93–8.

[119] Rodriguez-Galindo C, Billups CA, Kun LE, et al. Survival after recurrence of Ewing tumors: the St. Jude Children's Research Hospital Experience, 1979–1999. Cancer 2002;94:561–9.

[120] Pratt CB, Stewart CF, Santana VM, et al. Phase I study of topotecan for pediatric patients with malignant solid tumors. J Clin Oncol 1994;12:539–43.

[121] Tubergen DG, Stewart CF, Pratt CB, et al. Phase I trial and pharmacokinetic (PK) and pharmacodynamics (PD) study of topotecan using a five-day course in children with refractory solid tumors: a pediatric oncology group study. J Pediatr Hematol Oncol 1996;18:352–61.

[122] Nitschke R, Parkhurst J, Sullivan J, et al. Topotecan in pediatric patients with recurrent and

progressive solid tumors: a Pediatric Oncology Group phase II study. J Pediatr Hematol Oncol 1998;20:315–8.

[123] Frangoul H, Ames MM, Mosher RB, et al. Phase I study of topotecan administered as a 21-day continuous infusion in children with recurrent solid tumors: a report from the Children's Cancer Group. Clin Cancer Res 1999;5:3956–62.

[124] Furman WL, Stewart CF, Poquette CA, et al. Direct translation of a protracted irinotecan schedule from a xenograft model to a phase I trial in children. J Clin Oncol 1999;17:1815–24.

[125] Blaney S, Berg SL, Pratt C, et al. A phase I study of irinotecan in pediatric patients: a pediatric oncology group study. Clin Cancer Res 2001;7:32–7.

[126] Saylors III RL, Stine KC, Sullivan J, et al. Cyclophosphamide plus topotecan in children with recurrent or refractory solid tumors: a Pediatric Oncology Group phase II study. J Clin Oncol 2001;19(15):3463–9.

[127] Cornbleet MA, Corringham RE, Prentice HG, et al. Treatment of Ewing's sarcoma with high-dose melphalan and autologous bone marrow transplantation. Cancer Treat Rep 1981;65: 241–4.

[128] Jacobsen AB, Wist EA, Solheim OP. Treatment of Ewing's sarcoma with high-dose melphalan and autologous bone marrow rescue. Monogr Ser Eur Organ Res Treat Cancer 1984;14: 157–60.

[129] Herzig RH, Phillips GL, Lazarus HM, et al. Intensive chemotherapy and autologous bone marrow transplantation for the treatment of refractory malignancies. Proc First Int Symp Autologous Bone Marrow Transplantation 1985;1:197–202.

[130] Dini G, Hartmann O, Pinkerton R, et al. Autologous bone marrow transplantation in Ewing's sarcoma: an analysis of phase II studies from the European Bone Marrow Transplantation Group. Proc Fourth Int Symp Autologous Bone Marrow Transplantation 1988;39:593–9.

[131] Burdach S, Jurgens H, Peters C, et al. Myeloablative radiochemotherapy and hematopoietic stem-cell rescue in poor-prognosis Ewing's sarcoma. J Clin Oncol 1993;11:1482–8.

[132] Stewart DA, Gyonyor E, Paterson AH, et al. High-dose melphalan +/– total body irradiation and autologous hematopoietic stem cell rescue for adult patients with Ewing's sarcoma or peripheral neuroectodermal tumor. Bone Marrow Transplant 1996;18:315–8.

[133] Chan KW, Petropoulos D, Choroszy M, et al. High-dose sequential chemotherapy and autologous stem cell reinfusion in advanced pediatric solid tumors. Bone Marrow Transplant 1997; 20:1039–43.

[134] Atra A, Whelan J, Calvagna V, et al. High-dose busulfan/melphalan with autologous stem cell rescue in Ewing's sarcoma. Bone Marrow Transplant 1997;20:843–6.

[135] Lucidarme N, Valteau-Couanet D, Oberlin O, et al. Phase II study of high-dose thiotepa and hematopoietic stem cell transplantation in children with solid tumors. Bone Marrow Transplant 1998;22:535–40.

[136] Ozkaynak MF, Matthay K, Cairo M, et al. Double-alkylator non-total-body irradiation regimen with autologous hematopoietic stem-cell transplantation in pediatric solid tumors. J Clin Oncol 1998;16:937–44.

[137] Prete A, Rosito P, Alvisi P, et al. G-CSF-primed peripheral blood progenitor cells (PBPC) support in high-risk Ewing sarcoma of childhood. Bone Marrow Transplant 1998;22:S21–3.

[138] Czyzewski EAD, Goldman S, Mundt AJ, et al. Radiation therapy for consolidation of metastatic or recurrent sarcomas in children treated with intensive chemotherapy and stem cell rescue: a feasibility study. Int J Radiat Oncol Biol Phys 1999;44:569–77.

[139] Perentesis J, Katsanis E, DeFor T, et al. Autologous stem cell transplantation for high-risk pediatric solid tumors. Bone Marrow Transplant 1999;24:609–15.

[140] Burdach S, van Kaick B, Laws HJ, et al. Allogeneic and autologous stem-cell transplantation in advanced Ewing tumors. An update after long-term follow-up from two centers of the European Intergroup Study EICESS. Ann Oncol 2000;11:1451–62.

[141] Horowitz ME, Kinsella TJ, Wexler LH, et al. Total-body irradiation and autologous bone marrow transplant in the treatment of high-risk Ewing's sarcoma and rhabdomyosarcoma. J Clin Oncol 1993;11:1911–8.

[142] Meyers PA, Krailo MD, Ladanyi M, et al. High-dose melphalan, etoposide, total-body irra-

diation, and autologous stem-cell reconstitution as consolidation therapy for high-risk Ewing's sarcoma does not improve prognosis. J Clin Oncol 2001;19:2812–20.

[143] Miser JS, Krailo M, Meyers P, et al. Metastatic Ewing's sarcoma (ES) and primitive neuroectodermal tumor (PNET) of bone: failure of new regimens to improve outcome [abstract]. Proc Am Soc Clin Oncol 1996;15:467.

[144] Kushner BH, Meyers PA. How effective is dose-intensive/myeloablative therapy against Ewing's sarcoma/primitive neuroectodermal tumor metastatic to bone or bone marrow? The Memorial Sloan-Kettering Experience and a literature review. J Clin Oncol 2001;19:870–80.

[145] Barker LM, Pendergrass TW, Sanders JE, et al. Survival after recurrence of Ewing's sarcoma family of tumors. J Clin Oncol, in press.

[146] Ladenstein R, Lasset C, Pinkerton R, et al. Impact of megatherapy in children with high-risk Ewing's tumours in complete remission: a report from the EBMT solid tumor registry. Bone Marrow Transplant 1995;15:697–705.

[147] Ladenstein R, Hartmann O, Pinkerton R, et al. A multivariate and matched pair analysis on high-risk Ewing tumor (ET) patients treated by megatherapy (MGT) and stem cell reinfusion (SCR) in Europe [abstract]. Proc Am Soc Clin Oncol 1999;18:555.

[148] Leung W, Chen AR, Klann RC, et al. Frequent detection of tumor cells in hematopoietic grafts in neuroblastoma and Ewing's sarcoma. Bone Marrow Transplant 1998;22:971–9.

[149] Bergan R, Hakim F, Schwartz GN, et al. Electroporation of synthetic oligodeoxynucleotides: a novel technique for ex-vivo bone marrow purging. Blood 1996;88:731–41.

[150] Merino M, Navid F, Christensen B, et al. Immunomagnetic purging of Ewing's sarcoma from blood: quantitation by real-time PCR [abstract]. Proc Am Soc Clin Oncol 2000;19:593.

[151] Disis ML, Cheever MA. Oncogenic proteins as tumor antigens. Curr Opin Immunol 1996;8: 634–42.

[152] Champlin R, Khouri I, Komblau S, et al. Reinventing bone marrow transplantation. Nonmyeloablative preparative regimens and induction of graft-vs-malignancy effect. Oncology 1999;13:621–8.

[153] Childs RW, Clave E, Tisdale J, et al. Successful treatment of metastatic renal cell carcinoma with a nonmyeloablative allogeneic peripheral-blood progenitor-cell transplant: evidence for a graft-versus-tumor effect. J Clin Oncol 1999;17:2044–50.

[154] Staege MS, Hansen G, Baersch G, et al. Functional and molecular characterization of interleukin-2 transgenic Ewing tumor cells for in vivo immunotherapy. Pediatr Blood Cancer 2004;43(1):23–34.

[155] Burdach S, Nurnberger W, Laws HJ, et al. Myeloablative therapy, stem cell rescue and gene transfer in advanced Ewing tumors. Bone Marrow Transplant 1996;18:S67–8.

[156] Ladenstein R, Peters C, Zoubek A, et al. The role of megatherapy (MGT) followed by stem cell rescue (SCR) in high risk Ewing tumors (ET). 11 years single center experience [abstract]. Med Pediatr Oncol 1996;27:237.

[157] Emminger W, Emminger-Schmidmeier W, Peters C, et al. Is treatment intensification by adding etoposide and carboplatin to fractionated total body irradiation and melphalan acceptable in children with solid tumors with respect to toxicity? Bone Marrow Transplant 1991; 8:119–23.

[158] Dunst J, Ahrens S, Paulussen M, et al. Second malignancies after treatment for Ewing's sarcoma: a report of the CESS-studies. Int J Radiat Oncol Biol Phys 1998;42(2):379–84.

[159] Paulussen M, Ahrens S, Lehnert M, et al. Second malignancies after Ewing tumor treatment in 690 patients from a cooperative German/Austrian/Dutch study. Ann Oncol 2001;12(11): 1619–30.

[160] Fuchs B, Valenzuela RG, Petersen IA, et al. Ewing's sarcoma and the development of secondary malignancies. Clin Orthop 2003;415:82–9.

[161] Kushner BH, Heller G, Cheung NK, et al. High risk of leukemia after short-term dose-intensive chemotherapy in young patients with solid tumors. J Clin Oncol 1998;16(9):3016–20.

[162] Rodriguez-Galindo C, Poquette CA, Marina NM, et al. Hematologic abnormalities and acute myeloid leukemia in children and adolescents administered intensified chemotherapy for the Ewing sarcoma family of tumors. J Pediatr Hematol Oncol 2000;22:321–9.

[163] Neglia JP, Friedman DL, Yasui Y, et al. Second malignant neoplasms in five-year survivors of childhood cancer: childhood cancer survivor study. J Natl Cancer Inst 2001;93(8):618–29.

[164] Hawkins MM, Wilson LM, Burton HS, et al. Radiotherapy, alkylating agents, and risk of bone cancer after childhood cancer. J Natl Cancer Inst 1996;88(5):270–8.

[165] Smithey BE, Pappo AS, Hill DA. C-kit expression in pediatric solid tumors: a comparative immunohistochemical study. Am J Surg Pathol 2002;26(4):486–92.

[166] Ricotti E, Fagioli F, Garelli E, et al. c-kit is expressed in soft tissue sarcoma of neuroectodermic origin and its ligand prevents apoptosis of neoplastic cells. Blood 1998;91(7):2397–405.

[167] Druker BJ, Talpaz M, Resta DJ, et al. Efficacy and safety of a specific inhibitor of the BCR-ABL tyrosine kinase in chronic myeloid leukemia. N Engl J Med 2001;344(14):1031–7.

[168] Druker BJ, Sawyers CL, Kantarjian H, et al. Activity of a specific inhibitor of the BCR-ABL tyrosine kinase in the blast crisis of chronic myeloid leukemia and acute lymphoblastic leukemia with the Philadelphia chromosome. N Engl J Med 2001;344(14):1038–42.

[169] Demetri GD, von Mehren M, Blanke CD, et al. Efficacy and safety of imatinib mesylate in advanced gastrointestinal stromal tumors. N Engl J Med 2002;347(7):472–80.

[170] Chugh R, Thomas D, Wathen P, et al. Imatinib mesylate in soft tissue and bone sarcomas: interim results of a Sarcoma Alliance for Research thru Collaboration (SARC) phase II trial. J Clin Oncol 2004;22(14S):9001.

[171] Toretsky JA, Kalebic T, Blakesley V, et al. The insulin-like growth factor-I receptor is required for EWS/FLI-1 transformation of fibroblasts. J Biol Chem 1997;272(49):30822–7.

[172] Benini S, Manara MC, Baldini N, et al. Inhibition of insulin-like growth factor I receptor increases the antitumor activity of doxorubicin and vincristine against Ewing's sarcoma cells. Clin Cancer Res 2001;7(6):1790–7.

[173] Toretsky JA, Thakar M, Eskenazi AE, et al. Phosphoinositide 3-hydroxide kinase blockade enhances apoptosis in the Ewing's sarcoma family of tumors. Cancer Res 1999;59(22):5745–50.

[174] Toretsky JA, Steinberg SM, Thakar M, et al. Insulin-like growth factor type 1 (IGF-1) and IGF binding protein-3 in patients with Ewing sarcoma family of tumors. Cancer 2001;92(11): 2941–7.

[175] Hidalgo M, Rowinsky EK. The rapamycin-sensitive signal transduction pathway as a target for cancer therapy. Oncogene 2000;19(56):6680–6.

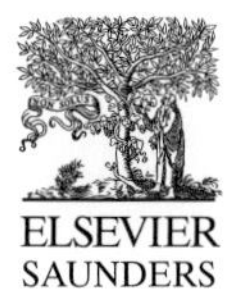

ELSEVIER
SAUNDERS

Hematol Oncol Clin N Am
19 (2005) 527–546

HEMATOLOGY/
ONCOLOGY
CLINICS OF
NORTH AMERICA

Sarcomas in Adolescents and Young Adults

Karen H. Albritton, MD

Adolescent and Young Adult Oncology Program, Center for Sarcoma and Bone Oncology, Dana-Farber Cancer Institute and Harvard Medical School, 44 Binney Street, Boston, MA 02115, USA

Sarcomas occur in all age groups, unlike the carcinomas that account for the vast majority of tumors of adulthood or the embryonal tumors of infancy. Although by total number soft-tissue sarcomas (STS) crest in the fifth decade of life, by percent of cancers for a given age, they peak in the child and adolescent, where they account for approximately 8% of all cancers (Fig. 1). Approximately 1800 individuals per year between ages 15 and 29 are diagnosed with STS in the United States (Fig. 2). STS is a large contributor to cancer mortality in this age group, because it has a worse prognosis than the more common cancers in the age group (melanoma, thyroid cancer, Hodgkin lymphoma, and germ cell tumors).

Adolescents and young adults (AYAs) with STS—defined here as patients diagnosed between age 15 and 30—are managed by both pediatric and medical oncologists and surgeons, further spreading out the care of a rare disease. In this review, I discuss relevant issues of tumor biology, adolescent development, and treatment variables that should be considered in the approach to the AYA patient who has soft tissue sarcoma. I also try to show that the traditional child–adult dichotomy of care does not serve adolescents and young adults well—in cancer or any other chronic disease, for that matter—and recommend clinical approaches to this population as well as new avenues for research.

Demographics of sarcomas in adolescents and young adults

For both rhabdomyosarcoma soft-tissue sarcomas (RMS) [1] and nonrhabdomyosarcoma soft-tissue sarcomas (NRSTS) [2,3], increasing age seems to be a negative prognostic factor, meaning that adolescents and young adults do worse than the average STS patient a pediatric oncologist sees but better than the

E-mail address: Karen_Albritton@dfci.harvard.edu

0889-8588/05/$ – see front matter
doi:10.1016/j.hoc.2005.03.007

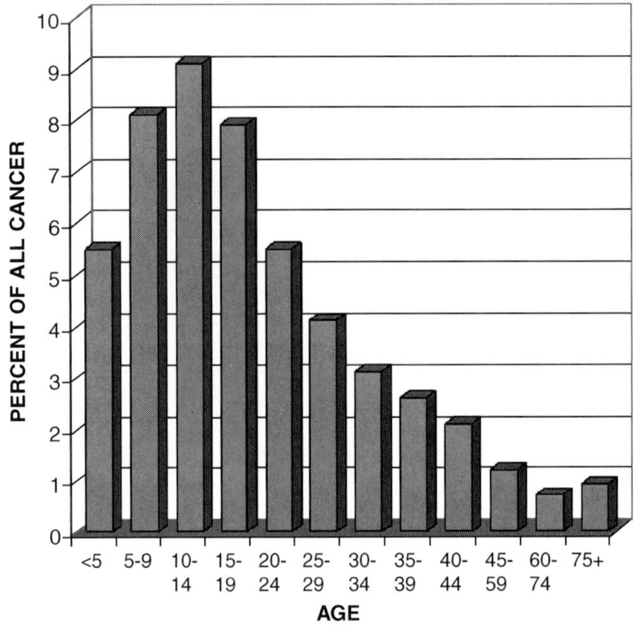

Fig. 1. Percentage of all cancers that are non-Kaposi soft tissue sarcoma, by patient age, from 1975 to 1999. (*Data from* the Surveillance, Epidemiology, and End Results [SEER] Program. SEER*Stat Database: Incidence—SEER 9 Regs Public-Use, Nov 2001 Sub [1973–1999], National Cancer Institute, DCCPS, Surveillance Research Program, Cancer Statistics Branch. Available at: http://www.seer.cancer.gov.)

average patient a medical oncologist sees. This interesting incongruity, where perspective and culture shape reality, influences the practical approach to a patient, as well as the more global research agenda.

For localized RMS, the 5-year overall survival (OS) for young children is greater than 75%, whereas in adults it is only in the range of 20% to 40% [4]. For

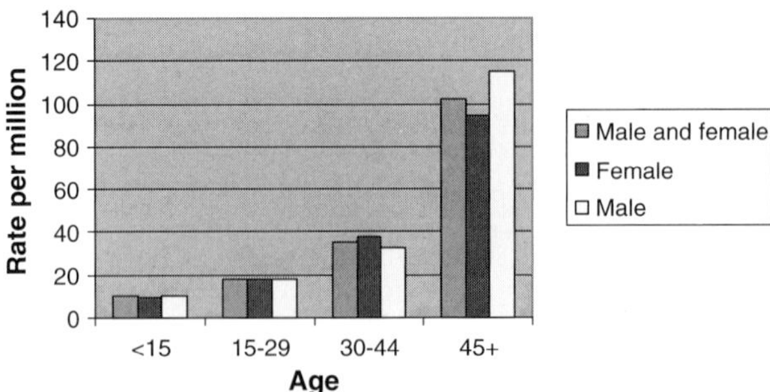

Fig. 2. Average annual new cases of soft tissue sarcomas in the United States, from 1975 to 1999. (*Data from* the Surveillance, Epidemiology, and End Results [SEER] Program. SEER*Stat Database: Incidence—SEER 9 Regs Public-Use, Nov 2001 Sub [1973–1999], National Cancer Institute, DCCPS, Surveillance Research Program, Cancer Statistics Branch. Available at: http://www.seer.cancer.gov.)

synovial sarcoma, Ocku's meta-analysis of 219 pediatric patients (52% of whom were 14 to 20 years) found that the risk of death increased 0.07 times for every year increase in age [5]. Age itself is probably only a marker for other variables of biology, patient characteristics, and treatment differences.

For AYAs with STS, not only is their prognosis poorer than for children, it does not appear to be improving (Fig. 3). In the two decades from the mid 1970s to the mid 1990s, the proportion of 5-year survivors among children under age 15 in North America with cancer has increased nearly 40%. Unfortunately, older adolescents with cancer, including those with STS, have not fared as well. For children who have STS, 5-year survival improved less so, approximately 17%; however, the 5-year survival for AYA STS improved only 7%. From 1985 to 1994, survival actually dropped for 15- to 19-year-olds from 70% to 63%. This was in spite of improvements in the survival for patients who have RMS (from 40% to 45% for 15- to 19-year-olds and 59% to 64% OS for 0- to 20-year-olds) (Fig. 4) [6].

Reasons for this lack of progress and worse prognosis include issues specific to this age group: some are inherent in the disease or the patient (differences in biology or intolerance of therapy), some are inherent in the system (treatment by physicians less familiar with the disease, delay in recognition of malignancy, lack of new therapeutic agents for sarcoma, lack of availability and participation in clinical trials), and some factors are influenced by the psychosocial milieu

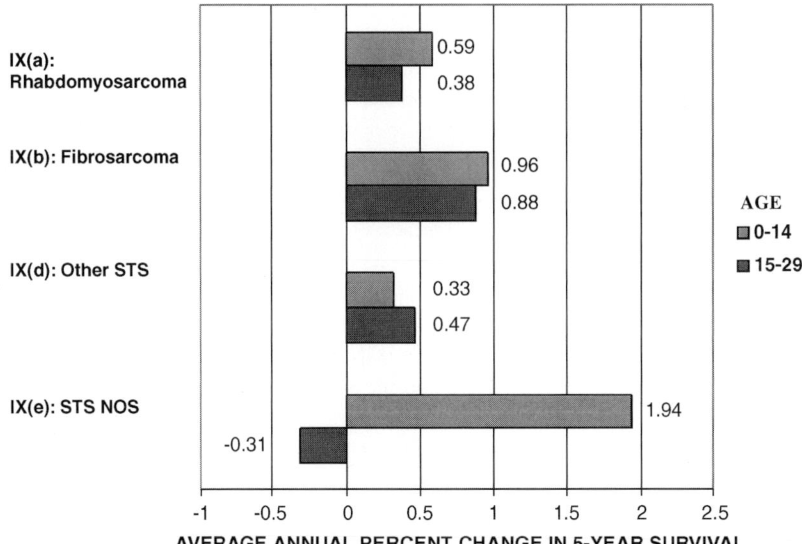

Fig. 3. Average annual percent change in 5-year survival by subtypes of soft tissue sarcomas the United States, from 1975 to 1998. (*Data from* the Surveillance, Epidemiology, and End Results [SEER] Program. SEER*Stat Database: Incidence—SEER 9 Regs Public-Use, Aug 2000 Sub [1973–1998], National Cancer Institute, DCCPS, Surveillance Research Program, Cancer Statistics Branch. Available at: http://www.seer.cancer.gov.)

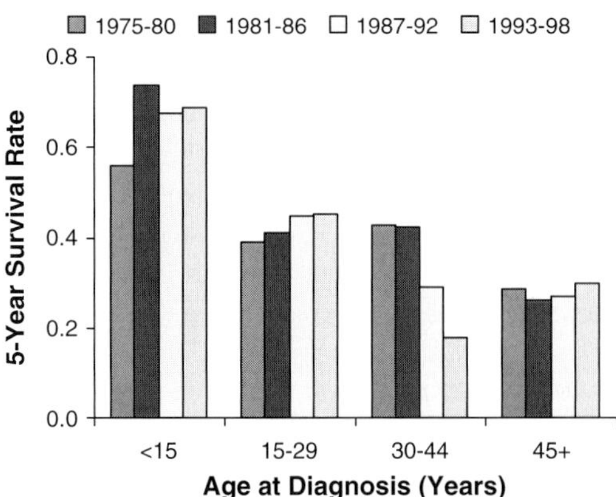

Fig. 4. Five-year survival rates for patients who have rhabdomyosarcoma and embryonal sarcoma, by patient age, from 1975 to 1999. (*Data from* the Surveillance, Epidemiology, and End Results [SEER] Program. SEER*Stat Database: Incidence—SEER 9 Regs Public-Use, Nov 2001 Sub [1973–1999], National Cancer Institute, DCCPS, Surveillance Research Program, Cancer Statistics Branch. Available at: http://www.seer.cancer.gov.)

of the patient (lack of medical insurance and financial resources, delays in seeking medical attention with symptoms of cancer, poor compliance with treatment, unwillingness to participate in clinical trials). Which of these might apply to the relative lack of improvement in survival for AYAs with STS? The answer is nearly impossible to extract from the data, given so mainly confounding variables, but several possible factors certainly contribute.

Issues in tumor biology

Different tumor classification systems in use for adolescent and young adult soft tissue sarcomas

In children, tumors are classified according to the International Childhood Cancer Classification system, based on morphology, which places all STS together, and then divides into RMS, fibrosarcomas (including malignant peripheral nerve sheath tumor, malignant fibrous histiocytoma [MFH], dermatofibrosarcoma protuberans [DFSP], alveolar soft parts sarcoma [ASPS], and primitive neuroectodermal tumor [PNET]), Kaposi sarcoma, other STS (including synovial sarcoma, hemangiopericytoma, liposarcoma, leiomyosarcoma, MFH and hemangiopericytoma/solitary fibrous tumor, malignant mesenchymoma, ASPS, chondrosarcoma and PNET) and unspecified STS. Rhabdomyosarcomas are the most common STS in children; because the other individual histologies are rare, they are often lumped together and called "nonrhabdomyosarcoma soft-tissue sarcomas," a term that sometimes perplexes medical oncologists not familiar with the demographics of sarcomas in the pediatric population. The pathologic classification system used for adult tumors, the International Classification of Diseases-

Oncology (ICD-O) [7], is geared toward carcinomas and therefore primarily organ-based. A category exists for tumors that arise in the connective tissue, but this would be misrepresentative, including germ cell tumors or carcinomas that occur in connective tissue and excluding sarcomatous tumors within organs. Therefore ICD-O data must be manipulated to classify by pathology subcodes to avoid misleading statistics.

Unique distribution of soft tissue sarcoma histologic subtypes in adolescent and young adults

The distribution of histologic subtypes of STS varies with age, with some virtually nonexistent either in childhood or in adulthood. Therefore the mixture of histologies seen in this age range is distinct from that in younger or older patients (Fig. 5).

RMS predominates in childhood, accounting for more than 60% of the STS in children younger than 5 years. In 15 to 19 year olds, RMS account for only 25% of the STS. In addition, the distribution of subtypes of RMS changes with age; although alveolar RMS accounts for 12% of RMS in children under 5, it is the subtype seen in 22% of adolescents age 15 to 19 (Fig. 6). Pleomorphic RMS is a subtype seen in older adults, and may biologically more closely resemble undifferentiated spindle cell sarcoma (MFH) than childhood RMS. It is equally uncommon below 15 and between 15 and 30. Experience with its lack

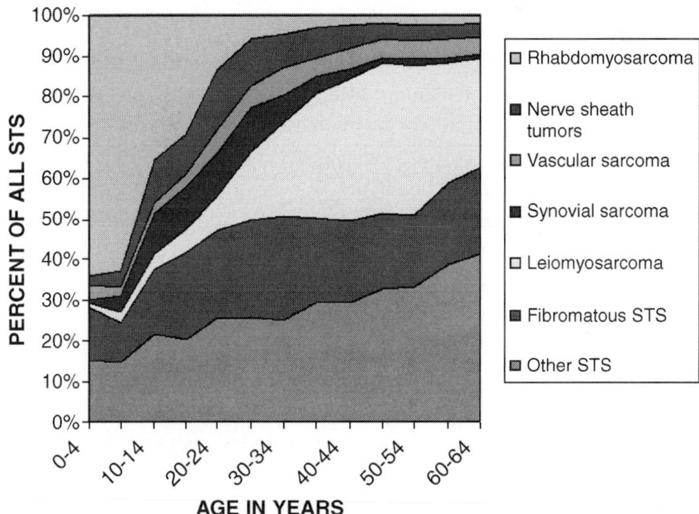

Fig. 5. Distribution of subtypes of non-Kaposi soft tissue sarcoma by patient age, from 1975 to 1999. (*Data from* the Surveillance, Epidemiology, and End Results [SEER] Program. SEER*Stat Database: Incidence—SEER 9 Regs Public-Use, Nov 2001 Sub [1973–1999], National Cancer Institute, DCCPS, Surveillance Research Program, Cancer Statistics Branch. Available at: http://www.seer.cancer.gov.)

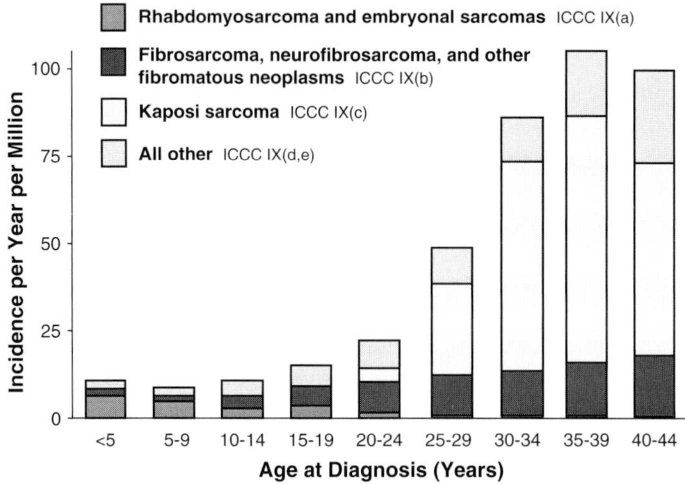

Fig. 6. Incidence of soft tissue sarcomas, per year per million, by subtype and patient age, from 1975 to 1999. (*Data from* the Surveillance, Epidemiology, and End Results [SEER] Program. SEER*Stat Database: Incidence—SEER 9 Regs Public-Use, Nov 2001 Sub [1973–1999], National Cancer Institute, DCCPS, Surveillance Research Program, Cancer Statistics Branch. Available at: http://www.seer.cancer.gov.)

of chemosensitivity and poor prognosis in older adults may unfairly bias adult oncologists against a curative approach to nonpleomorphic RMS in AYAs.

NRSTS, including synovial sarcoma, malignant peripheral nerve sheath tumor and fibrosarcoma, comprise only 40% of STS under age 5 before age 15, rise in incidence and account for 77% of sarcomas in 15 to 19 year olds. The Ewing family of tumors, including Ewing sarcoma (EWS) and primitive neuroectodermal tumor, when in soft tissue are pathogenically and therapeutically the same as when they occur in bone, and are not considered in this article. Similarly, Kaposi sarcoma begins to be seen in young adults over the age of 20 but has a different biology and management than the NRSTS and is not considered further. Several of the most common NRSTS in this age group bear individual mention.

Synovial sarcoma (a misnomer, as it does not derive from synovium or its precursors and does not necessarily arise near joints) is almost always a high-grade tumor of the extremities. Some pathologists contend a low-grade variant does exist, albeit rarely. The tumor has a characteristic t(X;18) translocation with two predominant fusion proteins (SYT-SSX1 and SYT-SSX2). Histologically it is composed of spindle cells alone (monophasic) or additionally, epithelial cells (biphasic variant, which tends to have a better prognosis). It seems to be more chemosensitive than some of the other NRSTS.

Malignant peripheral nerve sheath tumor (MPNST) is a spindle cell sarcoma with appearance and staining implicating neuronal origin (probably derived from Schwann cells). They are uniquely more common (~5% incidence) in individuals with neurofibromatosis type I (NF-1), a dominantly inherited disease. NF-1 patients have a mutated allele of the neurofibromin gene, resulting in hyperactivation of Ras, with resultant alterations in cell growth and differentiation.

In these patients, MPNSTs are felt to be a malignant transformation of large (plexiform) neurofibromas; when they arise spontaneously they also have somatic loss of N-1. These tumors are occasionally difficult to resect because of proximity to neurovascular structures. They are relatively chemoresistant.

There are two STS that appear in this age group that are unique in their biology and natural history: clear cell sarcoma (also known as melanoma of the soft parts) and alveolar soft parts sarcoma. Both have characteristic translocations [t(12;22) and t(X;17) respectively], are very chemoresistant, but can act very indolently. There are reported cases of these responding to interferon therapy, but once metastatic are almost uniformly lethal.

The broad remainder of STS in adolescents and young adults, including leiomyosarcoma, liposarcoma, fibrosarcoma, and undifferentiated pleomorphic sarcoma (or the controversially termed malignant fibrous histiocytoma, MFH) are early occurrences of these tumors commonly seen in adults and probably have similar biology and management.

Pathologic considerations for adolescent and young adult soft tissue sarcomas

There are several grading systems in use for STS, and pediatric and adult pathologists often use different ones, making comparison of results from different studies difficult. The French Federation of Cancer Centers (FNCLCC) system [8] and the National Cancer Institute (NCI) system [9] are most commonly used for adult STS and are based on a combination of mitotic rate, extent of necrosis, nuclear aberrations, and pathologic type of tumor. Pediatric studies have used the Pediatric Oncology Group grading system [10], which is similar to the NCI system, but future pediatric protocols plan on comparing this system prospectively with the FNCLCC system with the hope of moving closer to a common system.

Variation in biology of soft tissue sarcomas across age spectrum

For a given histology that occurs across the age spectrum, it is unclear if there is a spectrum of biology as well. Is there a reason to think that biologically an alveolar RMS in an 8 year old is different from one in a 25 year old or 55 year old? No studies (for example microarray analyses) have been done specifically looking at biologic variance in a given histology over age. What has been reported is a variance in presentation, with more advanced disease with advancing age, which may reflect biology but may reflect delays in diagnosis. Adults who have RMS tend to have larger, more invasive tumors with more lymph node involvement; 35% of adults are metastatic at diagnosis compared with 15% of pediatric RMS [11]. In a study of NRSTS from St. Jude Children's Research Hospital, STS patients between ages 15 and 22, compared with those under 15, had a higher percentage of tumors that were large and invasive, more with high histological grade and with metastases at onset [3]. Thus, with increasing age there appears to be increasing presence of adverse prognostic clinical findings that contributes to the poorer overall prognosis in these AYA patients.

Etiology of soft tissue sarcomas in adolescents and young adults

The cause of an individual STS is rarely known. However, there are certain known predisposing factors, of which genetics plays an important role. The Li-Fraumeni family of tumors includes STS. Likewise, retinoblastoma mutation carriers have an increased lifetime risk of an STS [12]. Radiation (eg, to the orbit for treatment of childhood retinoblastoma) increases the incidence even more, but STS incidence is increased outside the radiation port as well. Lastly, the incidence of STS in carriers of NF-1 is increased; the rate of MPNST is increased perhaps 300 times over that of noncarriers, but the rate of other STS is increased as well [13]. The prevalence of NF-1 in children enrolled into Intergroup Rhabdomyosarcoma Study-IV (IRSG-IV) with a confirmed diagnosis of RMS was 0.5%, approximately 20 times greater than that in the general population. The prevalence of one of these three predisposing genetic conditions in AYA STS patients is likely higher than in older adults, where sporadic or environmental causes prevail [14].

Therefore, the clinician should take a careful family history, perform a thorough physical examination, and consider genetic testing for suspicious cases. The advantage to knowing the result may influence the management of the patient and also the patient's family [15]. Mothers of children with STS have a higher rate of breast cancer, possibly due to germline p53 carriage [16].

Radiation-induced STS account for approximately 2.5% of all STS but probably occur in less than 1% of patients treated with radiation for a primary malignancy [17]. Lastly, although many patients relate a trauma to the area of sarcoma, a causative relationship has never been proven. Especially in physically active adolescents and young adults, this relationship would be hard to prove.

Presentation of soft tissue sarcomas in adolescents and young adults

The symptoms of an STS are the same regardless of age: usually a mass, beginning painlessly, but eventually growing to cause pain or dysfunction. Because of medical, psychological, economic, and social factors, older adolescents are at higher risk for a delay in diagnosis and can present with more advanced disease. In a study of the interval between symptom onset and diagnosis in 2665 children participating in Pediatric Oncology Group therapeutic protocols between 1982 and 1988, a multivariate analysis showed that for all solid tumors except Hodgkin disease, as age increased, lag time increased [18]. The reasons for delay in seeking medical care and obtaining a diagnosis are multiple. Adolescent and young adults have a strong sense of invincibility and may minimize physical findings. Out of denial or embarrassment, they may delay seeing a physician for symptoms. Once seen, clinical suspicion is low, and symptoms are often attributed to physical exertion, fatigue, and stress. Young adults are the most underinsured age group, falling in the gap between parental coverage and programs designed to provide universal health insurance to children (Medicaid and CHIP) and the coverage supplied by a full-time secure job. Lifetime uninsured rates for those who present for care peak for females between ages 15 and 17 (19%) and for males between ages 18 and 21 (24%) [19]. True uninsured rates are likely to be higher, as those who do not present for care may not do so because of lack of insurance [20]. Regardless of health insurance status, young adults and older adolescents have the lowest rate of primary care use of any age group in the United States. Many practitioners (eg, pediatricians, internists, nurse practitioners) receive little training in adolescent health issues and are not comfortable or willing to care for these patients [21]. It is unknown how much such delays and barriers might compromise outcome.

Psychosocial differences in adolescent and young adult patients who have soft tissue sarcomas

One of the greatest challenges and differences between the management of an adolescent patient and a younger or older one is in their psychosocial and supportive care. The adolescent and young adult is at a unique developmental stage, where the primary goal is establishing autonomy, separating from parents and family and succeeding at independent decision-making. The diagnosis and treatment of cancer disrupts and challenges this process. Some AYAs may revert to a dependent role and look to their parents for decision making and financial support. Others may try to continue to strive for independence and this can be stressful to the AYA and the parents alike. The physician must balance open and considerate communication with the patient and appropriate endorsement of parental discretion and authority.

For adolescents and young adults, the diagnosis of cancer is a devastating deviation from their plans, one that isolates and differentiates and defines them at a time that is all about defining oneself and fitting in. Many of the adverse effects of therapy can be overwhelming to an adolescent's self-image, which is often tenuous under the best of circumstances [22]. Weight gain, alopecia, acne, stunted growth, and mutilating surgery to the face and extremities as adverse consequences of cancer or treatment can be damaging to an adolescent's self-image. In particular, hair loss is cited over and over as a huge blow to the adolescent, especially the female, with cancer.

Their self-worth is developmentally dependent on peer group approval and usually measured comparatively. There are bars and milestones they have planned to hit including attendance of social events, grades, school performances, college and job interviews, early career achievements, and economic independence. AYA patients often feel behind, left out, or isolated. The cancer patient's issues are illness and death, whereas their peers are consumed by lipstick and homework. Cancer treatment for these patients must accommodate important developmental process. Consideration should be given to scheduling around sentinel events. Efforts should be made to minimize hospital admissions; with a motivated patient, willing home health services, or extended infusion room hours, most sarcoma treatments can be given in the outpatient setting.

Data suggest that adolescents are less compliant with oral medications [23]. Although currently most chemotherapy for sarcoma is intravenous, an increasing number of modern drugs are formulated orally. The treating team should work with the patients and their support (parents, roommates, spouses) to emphasize the importance of compliance, clarify who is responsible for the compliance (parent or child) and suggesting aids to compliance (pill boxes, calendars, pill counts).

This is a developmental period when sexuality, intimacy, and reproduction are central, but the young adult with cancer may feel or look unattractive, may be uninterested in or unable to have sex and may be made infertile by treatment. A feeling of impotence can pervade. Relationships will be tested by the strain of the cancer diagnosis and its therapy.

Lastly, a wide range of financial situations is seen in the older adolescent population. Some patients are still happily dependent on their parents. Some are just striking out on their own but, without a longstanding job or savings, may have to return to dependence on parents or get public assistance. Others are trying to begin a career but long work absences threaten their job security or growth. Older adolescent and young adult patients incur high medical bills at a time in life when they may least be able to afford them. Future insurability is certainly a stressful issue for all these patients.

Medical professionals caring for the adolescents and young adults may be used to the psychosocial problems more common in either younger children or older adults. Extra effort, including patient and family support groups specifically geared to this age bracket, should be made to uncover and address these needs, to increase compliance, reduce stress, and improve the quality of life during cancer therapy. Psychological or psychiatric support is often needed and prescription of antidepressants for situational depression may be beneficial. Although historically there has been a dearth of studies that address these issues [24], newer publications provide substantive management advice [25–32].

Issues in the treatment of adolescent and young adult soft tissue sarcomas

Low clinical trial enrollment

Given the great need for data to guide clinical practice, and its poor prognosis, STS should be treated on a clinical trial whenever available. Up to 65% of children under 15 are entered on clinical trials. In contrast, only about 10% of 15- to 19-year-olds who have cancer are entered onto a clinical trial [33,34]. Less than 5% of patients in their 20s enroll on a clinical trial. Rates for clinical trial participation of newly diagnosed STS are even slightly worse (Fig. 7). This dramatic deficit in clinical trials participation by AYAs may help explain their lower improvement in survival (Fig. 8) [6]. Some evidence indicates that AYAs who participate in clinical trials have more favorable outcomes than those who do not [35,36]. More importantly, a lack of participation by AYAs in clinical trials prevents us from being able to generalize the conclusions of those trials to this age group, and deprives the scientific community of the data to answer important biology and treatment questions.

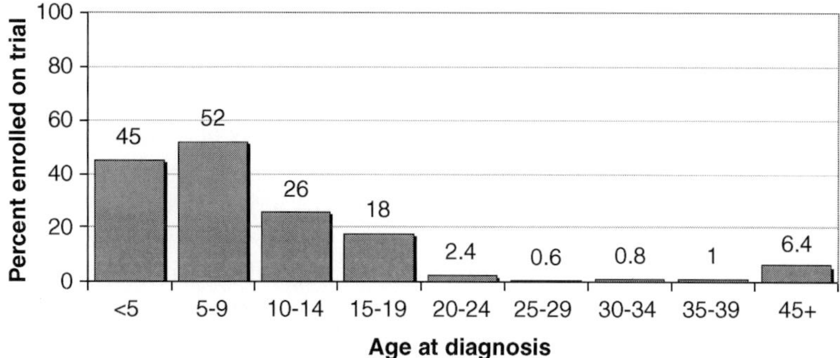

Fig. 7. Percentage of patients who have non-Kaposi soft tissue sarcoma (1993–1998) and are enrolled on National Cancer Institute clinical trials (1997–2001), by patient age. (*Data from* the Surveillance, Epidemiology, and End Results [SEER] Program. SEER*Stat Database: Incidence—SEER 9 Regs Public-Use, Aug 2000 Sub [1973–1998], National Cancer Institute, DCCPS, Surveillance Research Program, Cancer Statistics Branch. Available at: http://www.seer.cancer.gov. *Accrual data* from the Cancer Therapy Evaluation Program, National Cancer Institute. Available at: http://www.ctep.cancer.gov.)

Lack of specific trials for adolescents and young adults

One reason AYA sarcoma patients are not enrolling on clinical trial because there are no specific trials available. Indeed when a tumor is rare to start with and then the pool of patients is split between the adult oncologists and the pediatric oncologists, there is little academic critical mass to instigate such trials. This is further complicated by the relative lack of novel agents being tested in the pediatric sarcoma population. Trials specifically for RMS have been run by the IRSG of pediatric oncologists and until recently had an upper age limit of 21; in

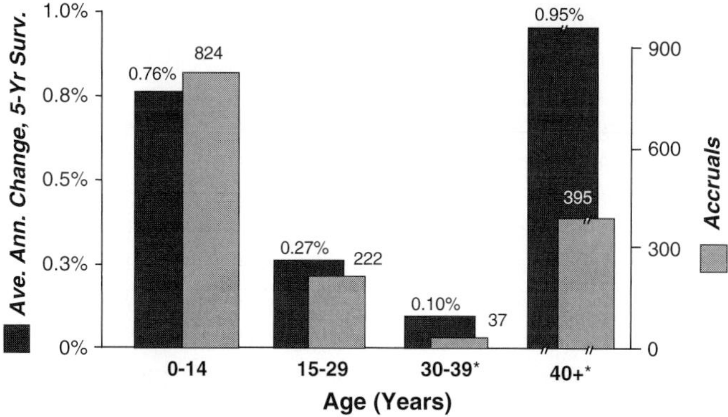

Fig. 8. Average annual percent change in 5-year survival rates (1975–1998) for patients who have non-Kaposi soft tissue sarcomas versus clinical trial accruals (1997–2001), by patient age. (*Data from* the Surveillance, Epidemiology, and End Results [SEER] Program. SEER*Stat Database: Incidence—SEER 9 Regs Public-Use, Aug 2000 Sub [1973–1998], National Cancer Institute, DCCPS, Surveillance Research Program, Cancer Statistics Branch. Available at: http://www.seer.cancer.gov.)

2002, this was changed to 50 years of age. There are still logistical barriers that keep older patients from entering the trials though, because the older patients are not seen by Children's Oncology Group (COG) investigators or at COG institutions. There have only been three prospective trials of pediatric NRSTS in the United States, enrolling fewer than 200 children and adolescents [37–39]. In adults, a few institutional or cooperative group trials for STS have been run in the last quarter century.

To cast the net widely, and without scientific rationale to the contrary, all ages and histologies of STS have been lumped together in these trials, so that little can be said about whether STS in younger patients should be managed differently. If all histologies of STS are lumped together in trials, the histologic variability gets lost, so that differences in survival by age may be a difference in the distribution of "bad actor" sarcomas. Recent collaborative efforts between several adult institutions and cooperative groups, including collaborations that include the COG, should finally allow studies that can be histology specific and that may allow studies specifically for young adults with sarcoma (similar to the approach in leukemia that opens separate trials for those younger and older than 60).

Effect of treating physician and location of treatment

For adolescents and young adults caught between the cultures of pediatric and medical oncology, treatment may vary a great deal, depending on the training, expertise, and cultural bias of the treating oncologist and the location of treatment and availability of clinical trials.

As is true of the care of adolescents in other nononcologic specialties, there are no "rules" that govern whether an adolescent is seen and treated by a pediatric oncologist or an adult oncologist [40]. Currently, the choice of specialist is made haphazardly and probably depends on the judgment of the referring physician. In contradistinction to children and early adolescents, who are nearly always seen by pediatricians, older adolescents are seen by a breadth of specialists for their presenting symptoms of cancer [41]. Several studies have shown that although children under age 10 are almost always then referred to a pediatric oncologist, the percent drops off between age 10 and 15, and the minority (approximately one third) of 15 to19 year olds are seen by pediatric specialists or centers [40]. Research is only now being done to ascertain the reasons for this practice pattern. The only survey of medical oncologists on the subject had a poor response rate (29%) and concluded that medical oncologists believe that they appropriately treated adolescents as adults [42]. Without outcome data to guide practice (explaining what influences the outcome of an AYA patient and whether those elements are provided differently in the two settings), we can neither say referral patterns are inappropriate or make suggestions to improve practice at the other setting.

It is unclear if there is a single right answer to where and by whom the adolescent with cancer should be treated. A 1997 American Academy of Pediatrics consensus statement considered referral to a board-eligible or board-certified pediatric hematologist-oncologist and pediatric subspecialty consultants as the standard of care for all pediatric and adolescent cancer patients [43]. A wider consensus panel that included adult oncologists, the American Federation of Clinical Oncologic Societies, also concluded that "payors must provide ready access to pediatric oncologists, recognizing that childhood cancers are biologically distinct" and that the "likelihood of successful outcome in children is enhanced when treatment is provided by pediatric cancer specialists" [44]. However, neither of these statements defines an age cutoff for the recommendation. Many older teenagers like to see themselves as young adults, not children, and physicians, as seen by the survey mentioned previously, are not inclined to say otherwise.

The answer to which specialist is most appropriate certainly varies from case to case. Patients at any age who have a "pediatric" tumor, such as rhabdomyosarcoma, Ewing sarcoma, and osteosarcoma, will probably benefit from the expertise of a pediatric oncologist, at least in the form of consultation. Children under the age of 18 and their parents may benefit from the social and supportive culture of a pediatric hospital regardless of the diagnosis. Individuals between the ages of 16 and 24 may have varying levels of maturity and independence, and choice of physician and setting for their care should be individually determined. Pediatric oncologists may be less adept at a nonpaternalistic relationship with the patient (and potentially his or her spouse) and less inclined to consider issues such as sexuality, body image, fertility. Adult oncologists are more accustomed to dose delays and adjustments and may be less willing to be aggressive with dosing that can be tolerated by the younger patient. Adolescent patients are more verbal about their desire to receive treatment close to home, to maintain a "normal" social life, whereas younger children are more easily uprooted and transported by parents to centers at a distance. This may deprive adolescents the advantages of a tertiary care center, including expertise, experience, and clinical trial availability.

In the end, the decision should be based in large part on which setting will provide the patient with the best outcome. If these are equivalent, "social" or "supportive" factors should weigh into the decision. However, increasing data suggest a disparity of objective survival outcomes. For those malignancies that have been treated by both pediatric and adult oncologists, with approaches typical of their respective disciplines, comparisons have shown that the pediatric therapy has been more effective. Outside of STS, acute lymphoblastic leukemia, Ewing sarcoma, and osteosarcoma have been found to have better survival rates when treated with the pediatric treatment approach [45–48]. The data are being analyzed for STS as well.

Management outside clinical trials

Staging

The work-up of a suspected STS in an AYA should be the same as in other age groups and include staging with a chest CT and bone scan, MRI or CT of the primary and a biopsy of tumor. Compared with the diagnosis of cancer in children, the diagnosis of cancer in adolescents is facilitated by the older patient's ability to describe and localize the symptoms and signs caused by the malignancy and the greater ease with which biopsies can be obtained. Noninvasive imaging without the need for sedation, and minimally invasive surgery without general anesthesia are all available for patients in this age group, an advantage over younger children.

Staging systems for STS also vary between pediatric and adult cultures. The IRSG system is based on a postsurgical grouping system and on a pretreatment clinical tumor-node metastasis (TNM) classification, where T is defined by tumor size and confinement to organ. The Musculoskeletal Tumor Staging System relies on definition of compartmentalization and the American Joint Council on Cancer (AJCC) Staging system combines TNM and histologic grading.

Low-grade STS in AYAs, as in other age groups, are treated with complete surgical excision and consideration of radiation for positive margins. The approach to high-grade STS is more controversial.

Local tumor control

Surgery is the mainstay of therapy. Although improved surgical techniques allow limb salvage in most circumstances, occasionally amputations are still deemed the best method for local control. Amputations are more adaptively challenging for the adolescent or young adult than for the younger child and may be more psychologically difficult than for the older adult.

Radiation should be considered for large STS, either neo-adjuvantly (to reduce fields, and thereby late morbidities, and potentially aid respectability) or postoperatively. It should also be used for high-grade tumors with less than a compartmental resection. Adolescents are generally spared the adverse effects of ionizing radiation to vulnerable developing tissues. This is particularly true for the central nervous system, the cardiovascular system, connective tissue, and the musculoskeletal system, each of which may be irradiated to higher doses or larger volumes with less long-term morbidity and growth disturbances that limit radiation in the young child. Accommodating school or work schedules for the daily routines of radiotherapy, as well as the increasing prevalence of obesity has complicated radiotherapy planning and delivery in adolescents. Because of the longer years of remaining life, the issues of risk of secondary malignancy must be considered even more in the AYA patient than in the older adult.

Adjuvant chemotherapy

The benefit of chemotherapy for adult-high grade STS has been studied but remains unclear because of a lack of definitive randomized data [49]. Only one randomized trial of adjuvant chemotherapy has been done in pediatric NRSTS, and it showed no difference in 3-year DFS [37]. However, probably influenced in part by the chemo-sensitivity of RMS (and EWS), the pediatric oncology community has been inclined to use more adjuvant chemotherapy in addition to aggressive local control in the treatment of high-risk STS. Adult oncologists have been more nihilistic, based on the toxicities and poor prognosis of "all-comers," and off clinical trial, the use of adjuvant chemotherapy is less common.

The risk/benefit analysis may be slightly different in the AYA. The risk of toxicity is probably lower than in adults (given a lack of comorbidities and normal organ function) and one could hypothesize that the tolerance of equal toxicity may be higher. Although there are few data on the difference in pharmacokinetics of chemotherapeutic agents between the ages of 10 and 50, it is unlikely that there would be changes between the age of 15 and 30, an argument for treating all patients in this age group similarly. The possibility of chemosensitivity may be higher in AYAs, because the histologies more often seen in the AYA have higher response rates (synovial sarcoma, RMS). The data from the adult trials may not be relevant to the AYA STS patient because none of the studies had the power to analyze outcomes specifically for these younger patients.

Lastly, the very process of decision making, of weighing the pros and cons of chemotherapy, is different for this population. The adolescent or young adult may not be mature or informed enough to make the decision on his own. Yet, he is too independent (legally and developmentally) to have a parent or physician make the decision for him without his input. Also, a strong sense of hopefulness and future-orientation often contributes to the decision making for the AYA and family, sometimes weighting a choice toward adjuvant therapy in spite of negligible benefit.

Rhabdomyosarcoma

Ferrari et al [11] retrospectively analyzed 171 adult patients aged 19 to 83 (mean 27) with nonpleomorphic RMS to determine the prognostic significance of aggressive, pediatric-type therapy, which was defined as multidrug chemotherapy (cyclophosphamide or ifosfamide; doxorubicin, epirubicin or dactinomycin; ±vincristine) for at least eight cycles, surgery, and radiation for incomplete resections. The average survival of all patients was 40%, similar to the high end of other published adult studies. However, survival of the patients who received pediatric based therapy (given in 45% of 19- to 30-year-old patients) was 61% compared with 37% for those who did not. Also, the response rate to chemotherapy in the 59 assessable patients was 85%, which is much higher than that quoted for adult NRSTS and not dissimilar from that seen in pediatric RMS. This chemosensitivity allows for less morbid surgical approach.

Primary resection should be reserved for cases where a complete, negative-margin, nonmutilating excision is guaranteed; otherwise biopsy and neo-adjuvant chemotherapy are recommended. Although retrospective, this suggests that every effort should be made to treat adult patients with nonpleomorphic RMS as close to IRSG-derived regimens as feasible. In the United States, vincristine, dactinomycin, and cyclophosphamide (VAC) is standard therapy with current protocols testing irinotecan or topotecan for higher risk patients. In Europe, ifosfamide is typically used instead of cyclophosphamide; current protocols are testing early intense doxorubicin. Most AYA patients should be able to tolerate this level of aggressiveness, although it should not fail to be recognized that older adults may be considered for such therapy but are unable to complete it because of toxicities or co-morbidities not seen in younger children. Retrospective analyses are complicated by supportive care and monitoring differences, so that dose adjustments or delays may reflect differences in therapeutic approach rather than true differences in patient substrate. Alveolar RMS, a more common subtype in AYA patients, has been thought to require the addition of radiation even in completely resected cases, meaning more AYAs patients suffer the side effects of this modality as well.

Synovial sarcoma

The other STS for which some analysis has been done is synovial sarcoma, an NRSTS with its peak incidence in the AYA age group. Prognosis worsens with age [50]. As with RMS, older patients present with larger tumors [11]. There is a trend for adult synovial sarcomas to be monophasic, which has been associated with a worse prognosis. Ocku's analysis of 219 patients under age 20 who have resected synovial sarcoma found no clear impact of chemotherapy on survival [5]. Ferrari and colleagues performed an analysis of 255 localized synovial sarcoma patients ages 5 to 87. About half of patients received chemotherapy, and half of those received ifosfamide and doxorubicin or epirubicin. Only 21% of those 15 to 30 years of age received adjuvant chemotherapy, compared with 78% of younger patients. There was a higher metastasis-free survival rate (MFS) in those who received chemotherapy, regardless of age, and especially in those who had tumors greater than 5 cm in size (MFS 47% versus 27%) [51].

Late effects

The quality of life is generally poor for the cancer patient during the period of active therapy. The acute and delayed toxic effects of cancer therapy are undeniably among the worst toxic effects associated with the treatment of any chronic disease. Acute nausea, vomiting, mucositis, alopecia, weight gain or excessive weight loss, acne, bleeding, and infection are to be expected. During treatment, delayed complications may be of less concern to patients in this age group (whose vision of the future is myopic) than to older adults and parents of younger children, but after therapy has been completed, such complications can be surprisingly disheartening, fearful, and can have terrible consequences. Examples include second malignancies, depression, infertility, avascular necrosis, cognitive dysfunction, or cardiac failure.

Remarkably little has been published on the quality of life of survivors of cancer during adolescence. Most of the reports are on adolescent survivors of childhood cancer, instead of survivors of cancer during adolescence, and it may not be appropriate to extrapolate. In one study, 41 adolescents who were evaluated at a mean age of 17 had completed treatment for cancer at 2 to 8 years of age. Of these, one quarter had poor global functioning or were considered counterphobic and hypochondriacal [54]. The subgroup of AYAs in the Childhood Cancer Survivor Study, a large cohort study of survivors of childhood cancer including STS diagnosed before age 21, may provide more insight into the issues of these survivors [52].

Many adolescent and young adult cancer survivors cite fertility as a primary concern that impacts the quality of their life. Yet most do not recall an adequate discussion of the risks of infertility or methods to decrease the risks with their physician at the initiation of therapy [53]. The provider must consider the estimated risk of infertility, the patient's maturity, and the need to initiate therapy immediately in framing the conversation about infertility and the options of germ cell preservation. Rates of infertility are very hard to predict for an individual and depend on gender, age, radiation dose and schedule, chemotherapeutic agent and dose [54].

Because of a decreasing pool of follicles, rates of amenorrhea and infertility are positively associated with increasing age of the patient at the time of treatment, so that the rates in adolescent females appear intermediate between those lower rates of prepubertal children and high rates in older women. Although permanent failure may not occur, there may be more subtle changes, which only become evident only with extremely prolonged follow-up of cancer survivors, for example, decreased libido and premature menopause (with resultant increase in risk of osteoporosis, heart disease, and so forth). Even if ovulation does return after the end of therapy, the patient should be counseled about the risk of premature ovarian failure, as it may narrow the window of fertility [55]. There are no established techniques to preserve fertility for women undergoing chemotherapy, but experimental approaches are being studied at specialized centers.

Rates of infertility appear higher in male survivors than female. Thankfully, fertility preservation options are more feasible and successful. Sperm cryopreservation should be discussed with all sexually mature males—usually collected via masturbation but epididymal aspiration and testicular wedge biopsy are also used. After both radiation and chemotherapy, spermatogenesis may return after years of apparent azoospermia and adolescents should be counseled regarding this possibility [56].

Other late effects depend on the types of therapy received. Some common ones seen include cardiac insufficiency due to anthracyclines, renal insufficiency due to alkylators, and secondary malignancies due to chemotherapy (especially leukemias) and radiation (especially sarcomas). Patients should be educated by their oncologists about the possibility of these and the primary care physician and oncologist should coordinate monitoring for them. Although guidelines for follow-up of cancer patients treated during adolescence and young adulthood have not been generated, a comprehensive document prepared by the Children's Oncology Group for childhood cancer survivors is probably mostly applicable, and is available on the Web site http://www.survivorshipguidelines.org. The follow-up for adolescent and young adult cancer patients is made difficult not only by their sense of invincibility (especially after surviving cancer) and their mediocre compliance but, if they have received care in a pediatric system, their inevitable transition to adult services [56].

Summary

The AYA STS patient is a complex challenge. Providers must contend with delays in diagnosis, confusing classification, grading and staging systems, challenging communication with patient and parent, and issues such as fertility, school, adherence, sexuality, and depression. The physician should consider host factors, physiology, and comorbidities in planning therapy. Lastly, one should seek out AYA and histology-specific data when available and be aware of problems extrapolating data from older adults or younger children. The future holds more promise than ever for AYAs who have STS. We look forward to more outcome data to elucidate the important factors influencing survival and quality of life for these patients, studies of the biology of tumors over the age spectrum, increased awareness of the benefit of referral to specialized centers of sarcoma excellence which have both pediatric and adult expertise, and an increasing number of clinical trials studying the STS that affect this age group.

References

[1] Joshi D, Anderson JR, Paidas C, et al. Age is an independent prognostic factor in rhabdomyosarcoma: a report from the Soft Tissue Sarcoma Committee of the Children's Oncology Group. Pediatr Blood Cancer 2004;42:64–73.

[2] Kattan MW, Leung DHY, Brennan MF. Postoperative nomogram for 12-year sarcoma-specific death. J Clin Oncol 2002;20:791–6.

[3] Hayes-Jordan AA, Spunt SL, Poquette CA, et al. Nonrhabdomyosarcoma soft tissue sarcomas in children: is age at diagnosis an important variable? J Pediatr Surg 2000;35:948–53.

[4] Raney RB, Anderson JR, Barr FG, et al. Rhabdomyosarcoma and undifferentiated sarcoma in the first two decades of life: a selective review of intergroup rhabdomyosarcoma study group experience and rationale for Intergroup Rhabdomyosarcoma Study V. J Pediatr Hematol Oncol 2001;23(4):215–20.

[5] Ocku MF, Munsell M, Treuner J, et al. Synovial sarcoma of childhood and adolescence: a multicenter, multivariate analysis of outcome. J Clin Oncol 2003;21(8):1602–11.

[6] Bleyer A, Montello M, Budd T, et al. Young adults with sarcoma: lack of clinical trial participation and lack of survival prolongation [abstract 3280]. Proc Am Soc Clin Oncol 2003; 22:816.

[7] Percy C, Van Holten V, Muir C, editors. International classification of diseases for oncology (ICD-O). 2nd edition. Geneva (Switzerland): World Health Organization; 1990.

[8] Coindre JM, Trojani M, Contesso G, et al. Reproducibility of a histopathologic grading system for adult soft tissue sarcoma. Cancer 1986;58:306–9.

[9] Costa J, Wesley RA, Glatstein E, et al. The grading of soft tissue sarcomas. Results of a clinicohistopathologic correlation in a series of 163 cases. Cancer 1984;53:530–41.

[10] Parham DM, Webber BL, Jenkins III JJ, et al. Nonrhabdomyosarcomatous soft tissue sarcomas of childhood: formulation of a simplified system for grading. Mod Pathol 1995;8: 705–10.

[11] Ferrari A, Dileo P, Casanova M, et al. Rhabdomyosarcoma in adults. A retrospective analysis of 171 patients treated at a single institution. Cancer 2003;98:571–80.
[12] Wong FL, Boice Jr JD, Abramson DH, et al. Cancer incidence after retinoblastoma. Radiation dose and sarcoma risk. JAMA 1997;278(15):1262–7.
[13] Evans DG, Baser ME, McGaughran J, et al. Malignant peripheral nerve sheath tumours in neurofibromatosis 1. J Med Genet 2002;39(5):311–4.
[14] Sung L, Anderson JR, Arndt C, et al. Neurofibromatosis in children with rhabdomyosarcoma: a report from the Intergroup Rhabdomyosarcoma study IV. J Pediatr 2004;144(5): 666–8.
[15] Strong LC, Stine M, Norsted TL. Cancer in survivors of childhood soft tissue sarcoma and their relatives. J Natl Cancer Inst 1987;79:1213–20.
[16] Moutou C, Le Bihan C, Chompret A, et al. Genetic transmission of susceptibility to cancer in families of children with soft tissue sarcomas. Cancer 1996;78:1483–91.
[17] Mark RJ, Poen J, Tran LM, et al. Postirradiation sarcomas. A single-institution study and review of the literature. Cancer 1994;73(10):2653–62.
[18] Pollock BH, Krischer JP, Vietti TJ. Interval between symptom onset and diagnosis of pediatric solid tumors. J Pediatr 1991;119:725–32.
[19] Mills R, Bhandari S. Health insurance coverage in the United States: current population reports. US Census Bureau P60-223, 2003. Available at: http://www.census.gov/prod/2003pubs/p60-223.pdf.
[20] Ziv A, Boulet JR, Slap GB. Utilization of physician offices by adolescents in the United States. Pediatrics 1999;104:35–42.
[21] Veit FC, Sanci LA, Young DY, et al. Adolescent health care: perspectives of Victorian general practitioners. Med J Aust 1995;163:16–8.
[22] Woo SY, Sinks LF. Neoplastic diseases. In: Shearin RB, Wientzen RL, editors. Clinical adolescent medicine. Boston: G.K. Hall; 1983. p. 97–115.
[23] Tebbi CK. Treatment compliance in childhood and adolesence. Cancer 1993;71(Suppl 10): 3441–9.
[24] Whyte F, Smith L. A literature review of adolescence and cancer. Eur J Cancer Care 1997;6: 137–46.
[25] Selby P, Bailey C, editors. Cancer and the adolescent. London: BMJ Publishing Group; 1996.
[26] Yarcheski A, Scoloveno MA, Mahon NE. Social support and well-being in adolescents: the mediating role of hopefulness. Nurs Res 1994;43:288–92.
[27] Young MA, Pfefferbaum-Levine B. Perspectives on illness and treatment in adolescence. Cancer Bull 1984;36:275–9.
[28] Manne S, Miller D. Social support, social conflict and adjustment among adolescents with cancer. J Pediatr Psychol 1998;23:121–30.
[29] Worchel FF, Copeland DR. Psychological intervention with adolescents. Cancer Bull 1984;36: 279–84.
[30] Nichols ML. Social support and coping in young adolescents with cancer. Pediatr Nurs 1995;21: 235–40.
[31] Novakovic B, Fears TR, Wexler LH, et al. Experience of cancer in children and adolescents. Cancer Nurs 1996;19:54–9.
[32] Rait DS, Ostroff J, Smith K, et al. Lives in a balance: perceived family functioning and the psychosocial adjustment of adolescent cancer survivors. Fam Process 1992;4:383–97.
[33] Bleyer WA. The adolescent gap in cancer treatment. J Registry Management 1996;23:114–5.
[34] Bleyer WA, Tejeda H, Murphy SM, et al. National cancer clinical trials: children have equal access; adolescents do not. J Adolesc Health 1997;21:366–73.
[35] Nachman J, Sather HN, Buckley JD, et al. Young adults 16–21 years of age at diagnosis entered onto Children's Cancer Group acute lymphoblastic leukemia and acute myeloblastic leukemia protocols. Results of treatment. Cancer 1993;71(Suppl 10):3377–85.
[36] Stiller CA, Benjamin S, Cartwright RA, et al. Patterns of care and survival for adolescents and young adults with acute leukemia-a population-based study. Br J Cancer 1999;79:658–65.
[37] Pratt CB, Pappo AS, Gieser P, et al. Role of adjuvant chemotherapy in the treatment of surgi-

cally resected pediatric nonrhabdomyosarcomatous soft tissue sarcomas: a Pediatric Oncology Group study. J Clin Oncol 1999;17:1219–26.

[38] Pratt CB, Maurer HM, Gieser P, et al. Treatment of unresectable or metastatic pediatric soft tissue sarcomas with surgery, irradiation, and chemotherapy: a Pediatric Oncology Group study. Med Pediatr Oncol 1998;30:201–9.

[39] Pappo AS, Devidas M, Jenkins J, et al. Vincristine (V), ifosfamide (I), doxorubicin (D), and G-CSF (G) for pediatric unresected metastatic non-rhabdomyosarcomatous soft tissue sarcomas (NRSTS): a Pediatric Oncology Group (POG) study [abstract 1508]. Proc Am Soc Clin Oncol 2001;20:378a.

[40] Albritton K, Wiggins C. Adolescents with cancer are not referred to Utah's pediatric center [abstract 990]. Proc Am Soc Clin Oncol 2001;20:248a.

[41] Goldman S, Stafford C, Weinthal J, et al. Older adolescents vary greatly from children in their route of referral to the pediatric oncologist and national trials [abstract 1766]. Proc Am Soc Clin Oncol 2000;19:440.

[42] Brady AM, Harvey C. The practice patterns of adult oncologists' care of pediatric oncology patients. Cancer 1993;71(Suppl 10):3327–40.

[43] American Academy of Pediatrics Section on Hematology/Oncology. Guidelines for the Pediatric Cancer Center and role of such centers in diagnosis and treatment. Pediatrics 1997;99:139–41.

[44] American Federation of Clinical Oncologic Societies. Consensus statement on access to quality cancer care. J Pediatr Hematol Oncol 1998;20:279–81.

[45] Stock W, Sather H, Dodge RK, et al. Outcome of adolescents and young adults with ALL: a comparison of Children's Cancer Group (CCG) and Cancer and Leukemia Group B (CALGB) regimens. Blood 2000;96:467a.

[46] Boissel N, Auclerc MF, Lheritier V, et al. Should adolescents with acute lymphoblastic leukemia be treated as old children or young adults? Comparison of the French FRALLE-93 and LALA-94 trials. J Clin Oncol 2003;21:774–80.

[47] Paulussen S, Ahrens S, Juerge HF. Cure rates in Ewing tumor patients aged over 15 years are better in pediatric oncology units. Results of GPOH CESS/EICESS studies [abstract 3279]. Proc Am Soc Clin Oncol 2003;22:816.

[48] Mitchell AE, Scarcella DL, Rigutto GL, et al. Cancer in adolescents and young adults: treatment and outcome in Victoria. Med J Aust 2004;180:59–62.

[49] Sarcoma Meta-analysis Collaboration (SMAC). Adjuvant chemotherapy for localised resectable soft tissue sarcoma in adults. Cochrane Database Syst Rev 2000;4:CD001419.

[50] Bergh P, Meis-Kindblom JM, Gherlinzoni F, et al. Synovial sarcoma: identification of low and high risk groups. Cancer 1999;85:2596–607.

[51] Ferrari A, Gronchi A, Casanova M, et al. Synovial sarcoma: a retrospective analysis of 271 patients of all ages treated at a single institution. Cancer 2004;101(3):627–34.

[52] Hudson MM, Mertens AC, Yasui Y, et al. Childhood Cancer Survivor Study Investigators. Health status of adult long-term survivors of childhood cancer: a report from the Childhood Cancer Survivor Study. JAMA 2003;290(12):1583–92.

[53] Thomson AB, Critchley HO, Wallace WH. Fertility and progeny. Eur J Cancer 2002;38:1634–44.

[54] Byrne J, Fears TR, Gail MH, et al. Early menopause in long-term survivors of cancer during adolescence. Am J Obstet Gynecol 1992;166:788–93.

[55] Howell S, Shalet S. Gonadal damage from chemotherapy and radiotherapy. Endocrinol Metab Clin North Am 1998;27:927–43.

[56] Oeffinger KC, Mertens AC, Hudson MM, et al. Health care of young adult survivors of childhood cancer: a report from the Childhood Cancer Survivor Study. Ann Fam Med 2004;2:61–70.

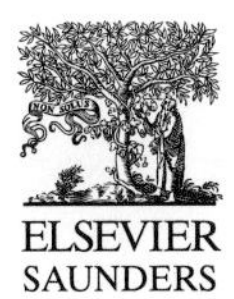

ELSEVIER
SAUNDERS

Hematol Oncol Clin N Am
19 (2005) 547–564

HEMATOLOGY/
ONCOLOGY
CLINICS OF
NORTH AMERICA

Gastrointestinal Stromal Tumors

Margaret von Mehren, MD[a,*], James C. Watson, MD[b]

[a]*Department of Medical Oncology, Fox Chase Cancer Center, 333 Cottman Avenue, Philadelphia, PA 19111, USA*
[b]*Department of Surgical Oncology, Fox Chase Cancer Center, 333 Cottman Avenue, Philadelphia, PA 19111, USA*

Gastrointestinal stromal tumors (GISTs) are the most common mesenchymal tumors of the gastrointestinal tract. They typically arise in the stomach, but can also be found in the small intestine, colon, rectum, and uncommonly in the esophagus and omentum. They are estimated to have an incidence of 10 to 20 cases per 1 million population, of which approximately one third are deemed malignant [1,2]. In the past, these tumors were commonly termed leiomyomas or leiomyosarcomas and had a reputation for poor prognosis. Disease commonly recurred in the peritoneum or metastasized to the liver. The mainstay of therapy was surgery with little documented efficacy of standard chemotherapeutic agents [1,3].

The outcome and prognosis for patients who have GISTs has changed with the identification of *KIT*, a type III tyrosine kinase receptor [4], as the biologic driver of the tumor [1,5,6]. During embryologic development, KIT is important for hematopoiesis, melanogenesis, gametogenesis, and mast cell growth and differentiation [7,8]. KIT is required for the development of the interstitial cells of Cajal (ICC), which are the pacemaker cells of the gut [9,10]. It is believed that ICC or their precursors are transformed by an oncogenic mutation in *KIT* [11,12]. Although most GISTs will express KIT, a minority will be negative for KIT or contain a wild-type gene for KIT [13]. Some of the wild-type *KIT* or KIT-negative tumors have been shown to contain *PDGFR-α* (platelet-derived growth factor receptor–α) mutations [14,15]. Mutations in *KIT* or *PDGFR-α* lead to constitutive activation of the kinases, resulting in continued growth and cell division, thus driving tumor growth. The presence of KIT and PDGFR-α recep-

This work is supported partially by a grant from the National Institutes of Health, RO1 106588-01.
* Corresponding author.
E-mail address: Margaret.vonMehren@fccc.edu (M. von Mehren).

0889-8588/05/$ – see front matter
doi:10.1016/j.hoc.2005.03.010

tors provide the rationale for testing of inhibitors of these tyrosine kinases. However, imatinib is ineffective in other cancers that express KIT, such as small-cell lung cancer, seminoma, and Ewing sarcoma, perhaps related to the lack of mutated *KIT* in these tumors. The efficacy of imatinib mesylate has significantly improved the outcome for patients who have metastatic and unresectable GISTs [16,17]. The agent is now being tested in the adjuvant and neoadjuvant settings. In addition, several agents are being tested for the treatment of patients who are refractory to or intolerant of imatinib.

Surgical management of gastrointestinal stromal tumors

Preoperative assessment

Percutaneous biopsy of a suspected GIST is not recommended because the tumors are often fragile, especially if large or there is extensive intratumoral hemorrhage or necrosis. Instead, endoscopic techniques for evaluation and tissue procurement should be considered for accessible tumors. In the initial evaluation of biopsy-proven GISTs, contrast-enhanced CT is the preferred imaging modality to determine stage of disease. Functional imaging with 18F-fluorodeoxyglucose positron emission tomography (FDG-PET) can complement standard CT by assisting with differentiation of benign from malignant tissue, necrotic scar tissue from active tumor, and nondescript benign changes from tumor [18,19]. Most GISTs demonstrate high glycolytic activity at baseline before imatinib therapy. Following the initiation of imatinib therapy, 80% of patients will demonstrate response based on PET images, which can occur within hours after a single dose of imatinib. Therefore, baseline PET scans should be considered before initiation of imatinib, or even surgical exploration if future treatment with imatinib is likely.

Primary disease

Clinically, GISTs range from small indolent tumors curable with surgery alone to aggressive cancers, but all should be regarded as having malignant potential. Complete surgical resection without rupture remains the primary treatment modality. The objective of surgery is removal of all gross tumor which, depending on factors such as location, size, and extent, may require subtotal, total, or even en bloc organ resection. Wide margins are not generally necessary for disease clearance. Systematic lymphadenectomy is also unnecessary because regional lymph node involvement is rare in GIST. In general, the standards for organ resection, organ preservation, and reanastomosis should govern the surgical resection techniques for GISTs. In contrast to other invasive intra-abdominal malignancies, gastric-based GISTs often protrude from the stomach, displacing surrounding structures. Complete resection can be accomplished in 40% to 60% of all patients who have GIST and in more than 70% of those who have primary, nonmetastatic disease [5,20–22].

Successful use of laparoscopic techniques for the resection of primary GIST has been reported in small individual series [23,24]. Tumors were small (3 cm), localized, and typically characterized as being benign or of low-grade malignancy. One group that used laparoscopic wedge resection to treat 34 patients who had submucosal tumors of the stomach, including 14 GISTs, reported no disease recurrences over a 5-year follow-up period. However, long-term data for patients who have undergone laparoscopic resection for GISTs are generally lacking, and the number of GIST patients in published cases or series is small.

Outcomes

The published results of surgical resection for primary GISTs have several limitations. First, most of the series contain few patients because the disease is uncommon, and therefore the experience at a single institution is limited. To compensate for the small numbers, investigators often analyze primary disease in conjunction with recurrent or metastatic disease. Results are also confounded by the inclusion of patients who have other intra-abdominal sarcomas (leiomyosarcoma in particular) because of the previous difficulties in the diagnosis and classification of GISTs. Furthermore, GISTs exhibit a remarkably wide spectrum of clinical behavior. Despite the recognition that certain morphologic features portend a more aggressive behavior, it remains difficult to predict the likelihood that a GIST will metastasize or recur following complete resection.

Very low risk GISTs have an excellent prognosis after primary surgical treatment, with over 90% 5-year survival. Evidence from long-term follow-up of patients who have undergone surgical resection of a high-risk GIST indicates that surgery alone is generally not curative. Before the introduction of imatinib, these tumors had an extremely poor prognosis even after surgical resection, with median survival of 12 months. As many as 85% to 90% had an adverse outcome, including recurrence, metastasis, or death [25]. In general, local recurrences or metastases develop in approximately half of patients who have potentially curative operations for GISTs, regardless of the site of the primary tumor, and 5- and 10-year survival rates after potentially curative surgery are 32% to 78% and 19% to 63%, respectively [26]. The median disease-specific survival for patients who have primary GISTs is approximately 5 years. Outcomes reported in recent studies are consistent with those in earlier series (Table 1).

Table 1
Major surgical series of CD117 + gastrointestinal stromal tumors

Reference	Patients	Site (%)	Localized disease at presentation (%)
De Matteo et al [6]	200	G (39), SB (32), C (15), O (13)	46
Pidhorecky et al [20]	71	G (45), SB (45), C (10)	56
Pierie et al [22]	69	E (1), G (39), SB (23), C (16)	51

Abbreviations: C, colonic; E, esophageal primary site; G, gastric; O, omental; SB, small intestinal.

Perforation or tumor rupture and the presence of residual gross disease are among the main factors portending an adverse outcome in patients who have undergone GIST resection. Incomplete tumor excision is associated with a significantly reduced disease-free and overall survival compared with complete resection. For patients who had complete GIST resections, 5-year survival rates of 42% have been reported, with 8% to 9% reported for those who had incomplete resections. In an analysis of 17 patients who had primary gastric stromal sarcomas, overall median survival was 19 months, compared with a median survival of 39 months after complete removal of the tumor. Tumor rupture eliminates the survival advantage conferred by complete resection of a nonlocally advanced primary GIST. In one study, it reduced the median survival from 46 to 17 months, which was comparable to the median survival after incomplete resection (21 months). Partial resection for palliative purposes is justifiable in patients whose overall performance status is good and who would benefit from the relief of symptoms related to obstruction or bleeding.

Recurrent or metastatic gastrointestinal stromal tumors

Outcomes in patients who had metastatic GISTs and in those who had GIST recurrence after primary resection were usually extremely poor in the era before imatinib; the median survival of such patients generally ranged from 6 months to approximately 18 months. After resection of the primary tumor, most patients subsequently recur. In some cases, tumor rupture can account for the recurrence, particularly if it occurs in the peritoneum. However, in most patients, recurrence develops after what seemed to be a curative resection. Strikingly, only 13 (10%) of 132 patients who underwent complete resection of the primary tumor were disease-free after a median follow-up of 68 months in the M. D. Anderson Cancer Center series [27]. The median time to recurrence is approximately 1.5 to 2 years. The first site of recurrence in GIST is typically within the abdomen and involves the peritoneum, the liver, or both. In the Memorial Sloan-Kettering Cancer Center (MSKCC) report, 27 patients who had complete resection of their primary tumor at MSKCC were followed up prospectively and had an assessable first recurrence. The first recurrence involved the peritoneum in half of the patients and the liver in nearly two thirds of the patients. Surgical resection may be beneficial in some patients who have GISTs who develop peritoneal recurrence. Unfortunately, what appears as limited intraperitoneal disease on preoperative radiologic imaging often turns out to be numerous nodules, if not frank sarcomatosis, at laparotomy. Recurrent tumors will be limited to the region of the primary tumor (25%) or located diffusely throughout the abdomen. It is uncommon to find extra-abdominal spread to the regional lymph nodes, lungs, bones, or subcutaneous sites. The liver is the sole site of recurrence or metastasis in approximately 40% to 50% of patients. As with primary GISTs, recurrent peritoneal nodules tend to rest on the surface of the intestine, omentum, mesentery, or abdominal wall and do not significantly invade the surrounding structures. Therefore, they can often be removed with limited resections.

Approximately half of patients presenting with first recurrence are amenable to surgical resection.

Results of surgical management of GIST recurrence or spread have been variable, depending on such factors as the stage of disease, tumor risk profile, and length of the disease-free interval after initial resection. In some patients whose primary tumor was a very-low-risk or low-risk rectal or anal GIST, locally recurrent disease has been treated successfully with total excision without further recurrence from 4 to more than 10 years. In their study of 239 GISTs, Clary et al [28] analyzed outcomes after resection of primary, locally recurrent, or metastatic GISTs. Complete resection was associated with improved disease-specific survival in all cases: 96 versus 26 months for primary disease, 49 versus 8 months for locally recurrent disease, and 39 versus 11 months for metastatic tumor.

Mudan et al [29] reported a median survival of 15 months after surgery for recurrent GIST. The longest survival was observed in patients whose recurrence consisted of hepatic metastasis alone. In this study, the only significant determinant of survival was the duration of the disease-free period between initial surgery and GIST recurrence, an indicator of the biologic aggressiveness of the tumor. In another study of 56 patients (34 who had GISTs or gastrointestinal leiomyosarcomas) who underwent complete resection for liver metastasis of sarcoma, an interval more than 2 years between diagnosis of the primary tumor and development of the metastasis was found to be a significant predictor of survival after hepatectomy. Complete resection of hepatic metastases was associated with prolonged survival in this study.

When the clinical presentation suggests that a patient who has recurrent GISTs might be a candidate for surgery, comprehensive diagnostic imaging is required for preoperative staging. In most cases, CT is satisfactory for the demonstration of GISTs in the liver, although MRI affords greater sensitivity for small lesions. PET is proving to be a sensitive staging tool and may be useful in identifying imatinib-resistant lesions. Complete surgical resection should be attempted in selected patients whose recurrent or metastatic disease is localized in a single site (eg, liver) or consists of low-volume, multiple-site lesions on the peritoneal surfaces. Resection of multiple intra-abdominal organs and tumor debulking are not warranted, except perhaps for palliation of localized bleeding or obstruction in patients whose performance status is otherwise excellent. Surgery for recurrent or metastatic GISTs is contraindicated in patients who have poor performance status and significant comorbid disease.

Unfortunately, resection of recurrent peritoneal GIST is seldom curative, even when all gross tumor is removed. Before the introduction of imatinib, adjuvant intraperitoneal chemotherapy using mitoxantrone was evaluated as a strategy for treating peritoneal recurrence of GIST following resection or debulking [30]. Nearly one third of patients harbored liver metastases in addition to their peritoneal disease burden. Treatment did not influence survival in patients who also had hepatic metastases; however, the median time to subsequent recurrence after therapy in patients who had disease isolated to the peritoneum was increased from 8 months in eight patients who had surgery alone to 21 months in 19 patients who had surgery and intraperitoneal mitoxantrone. The 2-year actuarial survival in these groups was 0% and 33%, respectively. This treatment concept has been largely supplanted because of the clinical efficacy of imatinib. Palliative use of chemoembolization for liver metastases has been effective in temporary control of lesions [31]. Newer approaches with radiofrequency ablation and or cryosurgery at the time of surgical debulking have also been reported [32].

Emerging approaches to combining imatinib and surgery

The possibility of cure afforded by surgery provides a rationale for using imatinib in conjunction with surgery. The role of imatinib as an adjuvant treatment to prolong disease-free survival and improve overall survival is being tested in several studies internationally. In addition, neoadjuvant imatinib to debulk tumors is also being evaluated in a phase 2 clinical trial led by the Radiation Oncology Therapy Group. Imatinib treatment in patients who present with inoperable malignant GISTs might enable them to undergo successful resection after a reduction in tumor size or spread. Pharmacologic debulking with imatinib may also be a strategy to optimize the timing of surgery and avoid emergency operations, with the attendant risk for complications, particularly in patients who have large GISTs that predispose them to hemorrhage or tumor rupture. In addition, neoadjuvant imatinib may allow a marginally respectable GIST to be resected, but requires close follow-up by the surgeon and medical oncologist for signs of response or growth on imatinib. Surgical resection of imatinib unresponsive lesions has been performed. There appears to be a greater operative risk in patients who have nonresponsive disease compared with patients who have some response to imatinib [33].

It is conceivable that if imatinib can improve the outcome of surgery, surgery might enhance the results of imatinib therapy. The extent to which strategies combining the use of imatinib and surgery in treating GISTs are feasible in actual practice awaits elucidation in clinical trials.

Medical management of gastrointestinal stromal tumors

Before targeted molecular therapies

GISTs are refractory to standard chemotherapy. Until recently, few studies separated GISTs from other sarcoma histologies. Edmonson and colleagues [34] conducted a trial of dacarbazine, mitomycin, doxorubicin, and cisplatin and enrolled two cohorts of patients: those who had leiomyosarcomas and those who had GISTs. The response rates contrasted sharply with a 54% response rate in leiomyosarcomas compared with 4.9% response rate in GISTs. In addition, 0% to 27% GIST response rates have been reported for regimens containing doxorubicin and ifosfamide 7% for those containing paclitaxel, and 0% for those containing gemcitabine [1]. One potential explanation for the lack of effectiveness of standard chemotherapeutic agents on GISTs is enhanced expression of multidrug-resistant proteins compared with leiomyosarcomas [35]. The limited response rates of these therapies were associated with poor survival in patients who had metastatic disease.

Targeted therapy: imatinib mesylate

The identification of *KIT* and *PDGFR-α* as the oncologic drivers of GISTs provided targets for therapy [3,36]. Imatinib mesylate, an oral tyrosine kinase inhibitor with activity against Abl, Bcr-Abl, KIT, and PDGFR [37,38], was hypothesized to lead to clinical benefit in GIST. Preclinical data demonstrated activity against wild-type and mutant forms of KIT [38,39]. Phase 1 testing demonstrated efficacy of the agent in GIST patients who had a maximum tolerated dose of 400 mg twice daily [16,40]. Dose-limiting toxicities were nausea, vomiting, edema, and rash, with the most common toxicities from GIST clinical trials summarized in Table 2. Hematologic toxicities were more frequent in stud-

Table 2
Toxicity profile of patients receiving imatinib

	Phase 1, N = 40 (4 non-GIST) [16]	Phase 2, N = 198 (24 non-GIST) [17,41]	Phase 3 (EORTC), N = 972 [42]	Phase 3 (United States), N = 458 [43]	
Side effect	≥Grade 2	≥Grade 3	≥Grade 3	≥Grade 3	
Nausea	18%	5%	3%	Gastrointestinal[a]	14%
Vomiting	18%	5%	3%		
Diarrhea	NR	5%	3%		
Edema	25%	5%	6%	Cardiovascular	9%
Rash	13%	10%	4%	Dermatologic	5%
Bleeding, including intratumoral	8%	6%	5%	7%	
Anemia	NR	10%	12%	Hematologic[b]	19%
Leukopenia	NR	3%	3%		
Granulocytopenia	NR	10%	7%		
Neutropenic fever	3%	NR	NR		
Infection	NR	NR	4%	4%	
Fatigue	NR	NR	8%	NR	
Dyspnea	3%	NR	4%	Lung	2%
Pleuritic pain	NR	6%	6%	Pain[c]	8%
Abdominal pain	NR	3%	NR		
Liver function abnormalities	NR	3%	NR	3%	
Anorexia	NR	3%	NR	NR	
Flu-like symptoms	NR	NR	NR	6%	

Abbreviations: EORTC, European Organization for Research and Treatment of Cancer; NR, not reported.

[a] Encompasses nausea, vomiting, and diarrhea.

[b] Encompasses anemia, leukopenia, granulocytopenia, and neutropenic fever.

[c] Encompasses pleuritic pain and abdominal pain.

ies of imatinib in chronic myelogenous leukemia (CML) likely because of leukemic cell involvement of the bone marrow in CML [44,45]. In addition, the frequency of bleeding in GIST patients was greater likely because of bleeding with tumor response, particularly in the early trials of the drug when many patients had multiple bulky metastases. Factors impacting on toxicity have been evaluated with low hemoglobin correlating with hematologic toxicity, and low albumin correlating with development of edema and fatigue. Higher dose was correlated with edema, fatigue, rash, and dyspnea [19].

The trials of imatinib rapidly proceeded from phase 1 to phase 3 because of the unprecedented activity of the agent and the need to treat patients who were without other therapeutic options [16,17,40,41–43]. The phase 1 trials tested 400 mg, 300 mg twice a day, 400 mg twice a day, and 500 mg twice a day, with the latter dose identified as dose limiting [16,40]. The US-Finland trial, initiated before the completion of the phase 1 trial, tested 400 mg and 600 mg [17,46]. Although over 100 patients were treated, the study was not powered to determine superiority of one dose level over the other. A second phase 2 trial conducted by the European Organization for Research and Treatment of Cancer (EORTC) evaluated 400 mg twice a day in GIST and non-GIST patients [41]. Lastly, the two large international phase 3 trials assessed 400 mg daily compared with 400 mg twice a day.

The compiled response rates (Table 3) are comparable in the phase 1 and 2 studies but have slightly lower response rates noted in the phase 3 trials. The phase 1 and 2 trials in patients who had GIST had partial response rates of 54% to 71%, with an additional 17% to 37% with stabilization of disease. Patients who had symptomatic bulky disease noted rapid improvement in clinical symptoms correlating with the loss of metabolic activity seen by FDG-PET scanning [18,47]. Objective responses by CT scanning were reported up to 1 year after starting imatinib. However, earlier indications of response can be seen using tumor nodule density changes [48]. What is clear from these data is that imatinib, although effective, does not lead to many complete responses. Despite this fact, most patients benefit from imatinib, with 79.5% to 91% obtaining objective responses or prolonged stable disease. An analysis of the US-Finland trial found that patients who had stable disease as their best response to treatment had similar survival to patients who achieved partial or complete responses (Fig. 1) [49].

Table 3
Response to imatinib in metastatic and unresectable gastrointestinal stromal tumors

Response in KIT + GIST	Phase 1, N = 36 [16]	Phase 2, N = 174 [41,49]	Phase 3, N = 1673 [42,50]
Complete response	0%	1%	4%
Partial response	54%	71%	45%
Stable disease	37%	17%	28%
Progressive disease	9%	13%	21%
Not evaluable	0%	4%	4%

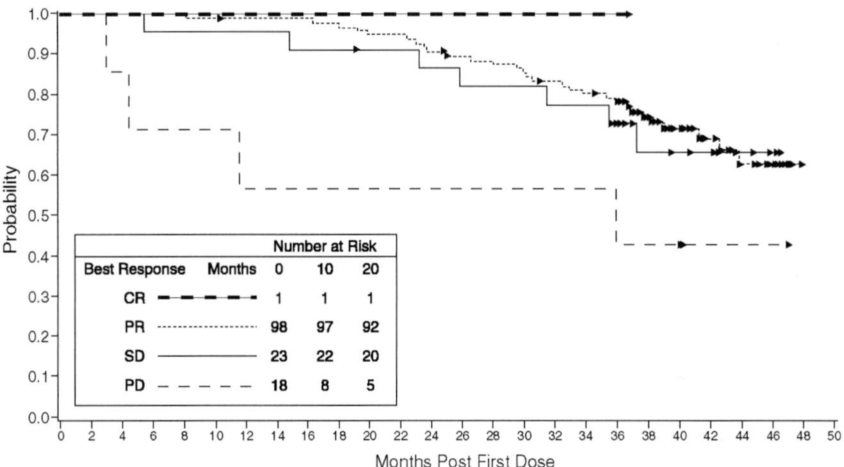

Fig. 1. Kaplan-Meier estimate of survival for patients treated on the US-Finland phase 2 trial. Patients whose response was unknown (N = 7) are not included. (Courtesy of Novartis, Basel, Switzerland; with permission.)

The phase 3 trials conducted in North America, Europe, and Australia rapidly accrued close to 1700 patients in 9 months. Both studies documented an increase in grade 3 and 4 toxicities in patients treated with 400 mg twice a day [42,43], although this was mitigated in the patients who began at 400 mg daily and then had their dose escalated to 400 mg twice a day at the time of disease progression [42]. Fatigue and anemia were more severe when switching from 400 mg daily to 400 mg twice daily, in contrast to neutropenia that decreased in incidence.

The lower response rates noted in the multicenter phase 3 trials are not unanticipated given the multiple investigators participating. However, the two studies arrived at slightly different conclusions. The North American trial, S0033, was powered to determine if one dose was superior to the other in terms of overall survival and enrolled 746 patients [43]. In contrast, the EORTC-led trial had as its primary endpoint progression-free survival and enrolled 946 patients. The EORTC-led trial documented an advantage to initiation of imatinib at 400 mg twice a day over 400 mg daily in terms of progression-free survival, without any difference in overall survival [42]. The North American trial found no statistical difference in the overall survival and progression-free survival between 400 mg and 400 mg twice a day [43,50]. The reasons for the differences in these conclusions are not clear. One possible explanation is that if the North American trial had accrued a larger number of patients, the same difference in progression-free survival would have been seen. However, there are other possible explanations. First, there may have been differences in the manner in which dose reductions and delays occurred between the two studies that affected the amount of the drug patients actually received in each study. Secondly, as discussed later, response to imatinib is correlated with mutation site in *KIT* and *PDGFR-α*. Therefore, differences in the distribution of the mutations sites in the low- and high-dose cohorts could result in a change in response rate and progression-free survival. Mutation analyses are being performed retrospectively and will be available in the future.

The length of imatinib treatment in patients who have advanced nonresectable or metastatic GISTs is the focus of a trial being conducted by the French Sarcoma Group [51]. This phase 3 trial randomized patients who have stable disease (SD), partial response (PR), or complete response (CR) following 12 months of treatment to stopping or continuing imatinib therapy. The primary endpoint of the study was to assess progression-free survival with secondary endpoints to assess overall survival and response to the re-initiation of imatinib in patients who discontinued imatinib. This study was the first to enroll patients who were not only KIT-positive by immunohistochemistry, but also patients who had KIT-negative GISTs with evidence of *PDGFR-α* mutations. The study was powered to detect a 10% to 25% difference in progression free survival (PFS) at 3 months. An interim analysis was performed in May 2004 on 48 of the 58 patients who had undergone randomization and for whom there was more than a 1-year follow-up. Of these, ten of the 25 patients whose imatinib was discontinued had progressed in contrast to none of the patients who were on continuous therapy. The median progression-free survival was 6 months in the patients who stopped imatinib, with 90% of the patients responding to the re-introduction of imatinib. Based on this interim analysis, further randomization was discontinued.

Determinants of response to imatinib therapy

Analysis of mutation site and response to imatinib in GISTs is relevant for a drug that binds KIT [4,12,52–55] and PDGFR-α [14,15] to inhibit their function. In vitro, all *KIT* mutations appear to be sensitive to imatinib, although mutations in exon 18 of *PDGFR-α* are not sensitive [56]. The largest reported series of clinical samples correlating tumor mutations with response comes from the US-Finland trial (see Table 3) [57]. Tumors were screened for mutations in the sites known to commonly contain mutations: *KIT* exon 9, 11, 13, and 17, and *PDGFR-α* exon 12 and 18. Of 127 samples, 93% percent were found to contain mutations, predominantly in *KIT* (95%) with few in *PDGFR-α* (5%). Most mutations were in *KIT* exon 9 or exon 11. Tumors with *KIT* exon 11 mutations had the highest partial response rates and survival, followed by tumors with *KIT* exon 9 mutations, followed by those tumors with no detectable mutations in *KIT* or *PDGFR-α*. There were too few patients who had *PDGFR-α* mutations or *KIT* exon 13 or 17 mutations to analyze.

Another factor that has become increasingly apparent in the management of patients who have GISTs and treated with imatinib is the differences in how this tumor responds radiographically compared with many other malignancies. There is a strong correlation with tumor response by FDG-PET scanning observed rapidly in the treatment course. Using standard response evaluation criteria in solid tumors (RECIST) criteria, achieving a partial response takes significantly longer. Lastly, response and progression can occur without evidence of significant change in the size of tumor lesions [48]. CT scans detect early changes in tumor density that precede the change in size of lesions. In addition, the growth of more solid areas can be detected within a lesion that represent outgrowth of a resistant clone of tumor cells. Recognizing the limitations of standard response criteria is crucial in the assessment of patients who have GISTs and are receiving imatinib.

Progression of gastrointestinal stromal tumors on imatinib

Clinical spectrum

There are two patterns of resistance to imatinib that are observed in patients who have GISTs. The first is a small group of patients who progress rapidly and never benefit from imatinib; the 9% to 17% of patients on imatinib trials who have progressive disease (PD) as their best response [16,17,42,43]. One possibility is that these patients did not have GIST, but another sarcoma with KIT expression. Many of the trials have incorporated expert pathologic review and genotyping of these tumors to minimize this possibility. In addition, response to imatinib varies based on the site of mutation.

The second cohort of patients are those who have been maintained on imatinib with an initial stabilization or response of their disease for more than 3 months, who then develop progression [16,42,43,58]. The median time to progressive disease is 18 to 24 months. This second group often has an increase in the size of some lesions, but not commonly all sites of disease; this is in marked contrast to the first cohort in whom all sites of disease progress. The cause of resistance at this time is not entirely clear. Mechanisms hypothesized to be of importance are the loss of KIT inhibition as a consequence of increased drug efflux or other pharmacokinetic factors, KIT amplification/deletion, or additional *KIT* mutations. Alternatively, KIT inhibition may still be present and then a second genetic mutation would be suspected. The 30% to 35% incidence of tumor stabilization/response to dose escalation in patients started at 400 mg daily of imatinib is indirect data suggesting that drug efflux mechanisms or pharmacokinetic factors may contribute to progression. To date, there are no reports of gene amplification of *KIT* or *PGDFR-α* as an alternate reason for the effectiveness of increasing drug dosage. There are increasing reports of metastatic lesions with additional mutations in *KIT* or *PGDFR-α* [59], and this appears to be the primary mechanism of resistance. It is not clear at this time if the development of secondary mutations develops under the selection pressure of imatinib or if these areas represent clonal outgrowth of a preexisting tumor cell with two mutations. Understanding the biologic mechanisms of resistance is important, as these patients will increasingly provide therapeutic challenges.

Clinical management of imatinib resistance

The initial question that needs to be assessed in patients who have progressive disease is the feasibility of surgical debulking of progressive lesions. Clearly, patients who are likely to benefit the most are those who have isolated progression and not those who have diffuse progression. Alternative palliative approaches include chemoembolization or radiofrequency ablation of liver metastases. Increasing the dose of imatinib in patients who have progressed on 400 mg daily is also an appropriate option, as it would be anticipated that up to 30% to 35% of patients would derive benefit with stabilization or response of their disease [45,50]. However, patients have had their doses of imatinib escalated above 400 mg twice a day without clear data on its benefits. Referral for clinical trial options is an additional option (Table 4). Lastly, for patients who are not candidates for the above measures and who do not qualify for experimental approaches, continuation on imatinib at a dose that is well tolerated is of benefit despite progression. Clinical trials that have stopped imatinib therapy before the initiation of alternate therapies have demonstrated increases in clinical symptoms and tumor flare by PET scan [60,61]. Thus, using imatinib until oral intake is no longer feasible is recommended.

SU011248

The agent with the greatest clinical experience to date is the multitargeted tyrosine kinase inhibitor SU011248 with activity against KIT, PDGFR, VEGFR (vascular-endothelial growth factor receptor) 1 and 2. Phase 1 testing of this agent evaluated various doses and schedules including: 25 mg, 50 mg, or 75 mg orally once daily for 14 days, followed by a 14-day rest period per cycle; 50 mg orally for 14 days with 7 days rest; and 50 mg orally for 28 days with 14 days rest. The latter schedule was selected for testing in the phase 2 and ongoing phase 3 trial in GISTs. Toxicities included: fatigue, nausea, vomiting, asymptomatic transient increases in lipase and amylase, uncomplicated neutropenia, hypertension, hand-foot syndrome, anemia, and bleeding at site of tumor biopsies. In addition, patients who had a history of coronary artery disease were found to have asymptomatic cardiac enzyme elevations.

Table 4
Therapeutic agents in clinical development for gastrointestinal stromal tumors

Agent	Targets	Phase of testing
SU011248	KIT, PDGFR, VEGFR	3
AMG 706	KIT and VEGFR	2
Bevacizumab	VEGF	2
BAY43-9006 (sorafenib)	Ras/raf, VEGFR	2
BMS-354825	KIT and Abl	1
RAD001	mTOR	1
PKC412	PI3 kinase	1

The phase 1 and 2 trials of SU011248 in patients who had imatinib refractory GISTs or imatinib intolerance treated 97 patients, 96% of whom had progressed on a dose of 600 mg or higher of imatinib [62,63]. Most patients had extensive metastases. PET scan noted decreased metabolic activity after 7 days of therapy, with CT scan responses evolving more slowly. To date, the PR rate is 8% with an additional 58% of patients having SD using RECIST criteria. The duration of tumor response had not been reached with a median follow-up time of 12 months. What was of particular interest was the response and clinical benefit observed in patients who have mutations that are less sensitive to imatinib, such as exon 9, wild-type *KIT*, and *PDGFR-α*, and those who have acquired mutations identified with the development of resistance (Table 5). This agent is currently in a phase 3 double-blind, placebo-controlled trial in patients who have imatinib-refractory GISTs or patients who are intolerant to imatinib. The primary endpoint of the study is to compare the time to tumor progression in patients treated with SU011248 to those receiving the best supportive care.

Other tyrosine kinase inhibitors

AMG706 is a tyrosine kinase inhibitor with specificity against KIT and VEGFR. An ongoing phase 2 trial is testing its efficacy in patients who have progressed on imatinib. BMS 354,825 [N-(2-chloro-6-methylphenyl)-2-(6-(4-(2-hydroxyethyl)piperazin-1-yl)-2-methylpyrimidin-4-ylamino)thiazole-5-carboxamide] is an Src-family kinase inhibitor. It has undergone preclinical testing in a mouse model of chronic myelogenous leukemia refractory to imatinib mesylate because of the structural similarities between Abl and Src, particularly in the setting of mutations seen in the Bcr-Abl gene in patients who became refractory to imatinib [65,66]. Animals treated with BMS 354,825 had a prolonged survival compared with untreated animals. A phase 1 trial of the agent has revealed responses in 31 of 36 patients who had imatinib refractory CML or

Table 5
Response to treatment based on c-Kit and platelet-derived growth factor receptor genotype

Drug	Mutation	N	RECIST response	Clinical benefit[a]
Imatinib [64]	Exon 11	85	83.5%	NA
	Exon 9	23	47.8%	NA
	WT KIT or PDGFR	9	0%	NA
SU011248 [63]	Exon 9	15	40%	80%
	Single PDGFR	1	0%	100%
	WT KIT or PDGFR	9	11%	55%
	2nd mutation exon 13 or 14	16	13%	56%
	KIT exon 11	7	0%	14%
	KIT exon 17	8	0%	38%

Abbreviation: NA, not available.

[a] RECIST-defined response + stable disease.

imatinib intolerance [66]. An ongoing phase 1 trial is evaluating efficacy in patients who have GISTs and other solid tumors.

Combination therapies

GIST tumors are vascular tumors. Immunohistochemistry has identified evidence of VEGF in GISTs, and patients who have metastatic tumors have been shown to have elevated serum VEGF (vascular-endothelial growth factor) levels [67]. A hypothesis based on the data of the SU011248 trial is that one important mechanism of disease control is the anti-VEGFR inhibition. Therefore, a phase 3 trial will be testing the combination of Bevacizumab, a fully humanized monoclonal antibody that binds VEGF, in combination with imatinib. In evaluating the pathway through which KIT and PDGFR signal, there are multiple other targets that could be inhibited. For example, RAD001, an inhibitor of the mammalian target of Rapamycin, is being added to imatinib [60]. RAD001 is a member of the phosphatidylinositol kinase–related kinase family in which a lipid kinase homology domain functions as a serine/threonine kinase to regulate protein translation, cell cycle progression, and cellular proliferation. The initial results have shown significant pharmacokinetic interactions between the two agents with increases in the serum concentration of RAD001 when given concurrently with imatinib, but no significant activity to date. Another agent that is being tested is PKC412, an oral staurosporine derivative that has activity against multiple kinases, including protein kinase C isotypes a, b, and g; KIT (WT and mutated); PDGFR-α and -β, VEGFR2, FGFR (fibroblast growth factor receptor), and FLT3 [61]. Pharmacokinetic studies of the combination of the effects of PKC412 when added to imatinib revealed up to 70% decreases in serum concentrations of imatinib. In contrast, when imatinib was added to PKC412, there was an increase in serum levels of PKC412 and increased toxicity. To date, three of 17 evaluable patients have stable disease. The phase 1 trial of this combination is ongoing to define the appropriate phase 2 doses.

Summary

The management of GISTs has undergone a rapid change since the demonstrated effectiveness of treatment targeting its molecular drivers KIT and PDGFR-α. This disease, previously only well controlled by surgery, was refractory to chemotherapy. Imatinib has altered the natural history of patients who have unresectable and metastatic disease, extending their lives significantly. Ongoing clinical trials are evaluating its benefit in the adjuvant and neoadjuvant setting to determine if therapy can improve survival and resectability of tumors. In addition, newer agents are being tested in patients who have imatinib refractory disease. At present, imatinib is the only agent that is approved for use in GISTs. However, it is likely that other agents will become available. Learning to correlate the site of *KIT* and *PDGFR-α* mutations with response will likely lead to the selection of a specific drug for a specific genotype.

Acknowledgments

We wish to acknowledge the assistance of Veronica Levin of the Fox Chase Cancer Center Special Services Department for the production of the figure in this review.

References

[1] DeMatteo RP, Heinrich MC, El-Rifai WM, et al. Clinical management of gastrointestinal stromal tumors: before and after STI-571. Hum Pathol 2002;33(5):466–77.

[2] Joensuu H, Kindblom L. Gastrointestinal stromal tumors–a review. Acta Orthop Scand 2004; 75:62–71.

[3] Miettinen M, El-Rifai W, Sobin LH, et al. Evaluation of malignancy and prognosis of gastrointestinal stromal tumors: a review. Hum Pathol 2002;33(5):478–83.

[4] Qiu FH, Ray P, Brown K, et al. Primary structure of c-kit: relationship with the CSF-1/PDGF receptor kinase family–oncogenic activation of v-kit involves deletion of extracellular domain and C terminus. EMBO J 1988;7(4):1003–11.

[5] Hirota S, Isozaki K, Moriyama Y, et al. Gain-of-function mutations of c-kit in human gastrointestinal stromal tumors. Science 1998;279:577–80.

[6] DeMatteo RP, Lewis JJ, Leung D, et al. Two hundred gastrointestinal stromal tumors: recurrence patterns and prognostic factors for survival. Ann Surg 2000;231(1):51–8.

[7] Broudy VC. Stem cell factor and hematopoiesis. Blood 1997;90(4):1345–64.

[8] Chabot B, Stephenson D, Chapman V, et al. The proto-oncogene c-kit encoding a transmembrane tyrosine kinase receptor maps to the mouse W locus. Nature 1988;335:88–9.

[9] Rumessen JJ, Mikkelsen HB, Thuneberg L. Ultrastructure of interstitial cells of Cajal associated with deep muscular plexus of human small intestine. Gastroenterology 1992;102:56–68.

[10] Huizinga JD, Thuneberg L, Kluppel M, et al. W/kit gene required for interstitial cells of Cajal and for intestinal pacemaker activity. Nature 1995;373:347–9.

[11] Chan JK. Mesenchymal tumors of the gastrointestinal tract: a paradise for acronyms (STUMP, GIST, GANT, and now GIPACT), implication of c-kit in genesis, and yet another of the many emerging roles of the interstitial cell of Cajal in the pathogenesis of gastrointestinal diseases? Adv Anat Pathol 1999;6(1):19–40.

[12] Hirota S, Isozaki K, Nishida T, et al. Effects of loss-of-function and gain-of-function mutations of c-kit on the gastrointestinal tract. J Gastroenterol 2000;35(Suppl 12):75–9.

[13] Fletcher CD, Berman JJ, Corless C, et al. Diagnosis of gastrointestinal stromal tumors: a consensus approach. Hum Pathol 2002;33(5):459–65.

[14] Heinrich MC, Corless CL, Duensing A, et al. PDGFRA activating mutations in gastrointestinal stromal tumors. Science 2003;299:708–10.

[15] Hirota S, Ohashi A, Nishida T, et al. Gain-of-function mutations of platelet-derived growth factor receptor alpha gene in gastrointestinal stromal tumors. Gastroenterology 2003;125:660–7.

[16] van Oosterom A, Judson I, Verweij J, et al. Update of phase I study of imatinib (STI571) in advanced soft tissue sarcomas and gastrointestinal stromal tumors: a report of the EORTC Soft Tissue and Bone Sarcoma Group. Eur J Cancer 2002;38(Suppl 5):S83–7.

[17] Demetri G, von Mehren M, Blanke C, et al. Efficacy and safety of imatinib mesylate in advanced gastrointestinal stromal tumors. N Engl J Med 2002;347:472–80.

[18] Van den Abbeele A, Badawi R. Use of positron emission tomography in oncology and its potential role to assess response to imatinib mesylate therapy in gastrointestinal stromal tumors (GISTs). Eur J Cancer 2002;38(Suppl 5):S60–5.

[19] Van Glabbeke M, Verweij J, Casali P, et al. Prognostic factors of toxicity and efficacy in patients with gastro-intestinal stromal tumors (GIST) treated with imatinib: a study of the EORTC-STBSG, ISG and AGITG [abstract 3286]. Proc Am Soc Clin Oncol 2003;22:818.

[20] Pidhorecky I, Cheney RT, Kraybill WG, et al. Gastrointestinal stromal tumors: current diagnosis, biologic behavior, and management. Ann Surg Oncol 2000;7(9):705–12.

[21] Crosby JA, Catton CN, Davis A, et al. Malignant gastrointestinal stromal tumors of the small intestine: a review of 50 cases from a prospective database. Ann Surg Oncol 2001;8(1):50–9.

[22] Pierie JP, Choudry U, Muzikansky A, et al. The effect of surgery and grade on outcome of gastrointestinal stromal tumors. Arch Surg 2001;136(4):383–9.

[23] Rothlin M, Schob O. Laparoscopic wedge resection for benign gastric tumors. Surg Endosc 2001;15:893–5.

[24] Otani Y, Ohgami M, Igarashi N, et al. Laparoscopic wedge resection of gastric submucosal tumors. Surg Laparosc Endosc Percutan Tech 2000;10:19–23.

[25] Heinrich M, Blanke C, Druker B, et al. Inhibition of KIT tyrosine kinase activity: a novel molecular approach to the treatment of KIT-positive malignancies. J Clin Oncol 2002;20: 1692–703.

[26] Lehnert T. Gastrointestinal sarcoma (GIST)—a review of surgical management. Ann Chir Gynaecol 1998;87:297–305.

[27] Dematteo RP. The GIST of targeted cancer therapy: a tumor (gastrointestinal stromal tumor), a mutated gene (c-kit), and a molecular inhibitor (STI571). Ann Surg Oncol 2002;9:831–9.

[28] Clary BM, DeMatteo RP, Lewis JJ, et al. Gastrointestinal stromal tumors and leiomyosarcoma of the abdomen and retroperitoneum: a clinical comparison. Ann Surg Oncol 2001;8(4):290–9.

[29] Mudan S, Conlon K, Woodruff J, et al. Salvage surgery for patients with recurrent gastrointestinal sarcoma: prognostic factors to guide patient selection. Cancer 2000;88:66–74.

[30] Eilber F, Rosen G, Forscher C, et al. Surgical resection and intraperitoneal chemotherapy for recurrent abdominal sarcomas. Ann Surg Oncol 1999;6:645–50.

[31] Rajan DK, Soulen MC, Clark TW, et al. Sarcomas metastatic to the liver: response and survival after cisplatin, doxorubicin, mitomycin-C, ethiodol, and polyvinyl alcohol chemoembolization. J Vasc Interv Radiol 2001;12(2):187–93.

[32] Patel S, Benjamin R. Management of peritoneal and hepatic metastases from gastrointestinal stromal tumors. Surg Oncol 2000;9:67–70.

[33] Hohenberger P, Bauer S, Schneider U, et al. Tumor resection following imatinib pretreatment in GI stromal tumors [abstract 3288]. Proc Am Soc Clin Oncol 2003;22:818.

[34] Edmonson JH, Marks RS, Buckner JC, et al. Contrast of response to dacarbazine, mitomycin, doxorubicin, and cisplatin (DMAP) plus GM-CSF between patients with advanced malignant gastrointestinal stromal tumors and patients with other advanced leiomyosarcomas. Cancer Invest 2002;20:605–12.

[35] Plaat BEC, Hollema H, Molenaar WM, et al. Soft tissue leiomyosarcomas and malignant gastrointestinal stromal tumors: differences in clinical outcome and expression of multidrug resistance proteins. J Clin Oncol 2000;18(18):3211–20.

[36] Coreless CL, Fletcher JA, Heinrich MC. Biology of gastrointestinal stromal tumors. J Clin Oncol 2004;15:3813–25.

[37] Buchdunger E, Zimmermann J, Mett H, et al. Inhibition of the Abl protein-tyrosine kinase in vitro and in vivo by a 2-phenylaminopyrimidine derivative. Cancer Res 1996;56(1):100–4.

[38] Buchdunger E, Cioffi CL, Law N, et al. Abl protein-tyrosine kinase inhibitor STI571 inhibits in vitro signal transduction mediated by c-kit and platelet-derived growth factor receptors. J Pharmacol Exp Ther 2000;295(1):139–45.

[39] Heinrich MC, Griffith DJ, Druker BJ, et al. Inhibition of c-kit receptor tyrosine kinase activity by STI 571, a selective tyrosine kinase inhibitor. Blood 2000;96(3):925–32.

[40] van Oosterom A, Judson I, Verweij J, et al. Safety and efficacy of imatinib (STI571) in metastatic gastrointestinal stromal tumours: a phase I study. Lancet 2001;358:1421–3.

[41] Verweij J, Van Oosterom A, Blay J, et al. Imatinib mesylate is an active agent for GIST but does not yield responses in other soft tissue sarcomas that are unselected for a molecular target. Eur J Cancer 2003;39:2006–11.

[42] Verweij J, Casali PG, Zalcberg J, et al. Progression-free survival in gastrointestinal stromal tumours with high-dose imatinib: randomised trial. Lancet 2004;364(9440):1127–34.

[43] Benjamin R, Rankin C, Fletcher C, et al. Phase III dose-randomized study of imatinib mesylate (IM) for GIST: Intergroup S0033 early results [abstract 3271]. Proc Am Soc Clin Oncol 2003;22:814.

[44] Druker BJ, Talpaz M, Resta DJ, et al. Efficacy and safety of a specific inhibitor of the BCR-ABL tyrosine kinase in chronic myeloid leukemia. N Engl J Med 2001;344(14):1031–7.

[45] Druker BJ, Sawyers CL, Kantarjian H, et al. Activity of a specific inhibitor of the BCR-ABL tyrosine kinase in the blast crisis of chronic myeloid leukemia and acute lymphoblastic leukemia with the Philadelphia chromosome. N Engl J Med 2001;344(14):1038–42.

[46] von Mehren M, Blanke C, Joensuu H, et al. High incidence of durable responses induced by Imatinib mesylate (Gleevec™) in patients with unresectable and metastatic gastrointestinal stromal tumors (GISTs). Proc Am Soc Clin Oncol 2002;21:1608a.

[47] Van den Abbeele A. F18-FDG-PET provides evidence of biological response to STI571 in patients with malignant gastrointestinal stromal tumors (GIST). Proc Am Soc Clin Oncol 2001;1444a.

[48] Choi H, Charnsangavej C, Macapinlac H, et al. Correlation of computerized tomography (CT) and proton emission tomography (PET) in patients with metastatic GIST treated at a single institution with imatinib mesylate [abstract 3]. Proc Am Soc Clin Oncol 2003;22:819.

[49] Demetri G, von Mehren M, Joensuu H, et al. Lack of Progression is the most clinically significant measure of a patient's clinical benefit: Correlating the effects of imatinib mesylate therapy in gastrointestinal stromal tumor (GIST) with survival benefits. Proceedings of the European Society of Medical Oncology. Vienna (Austria): European Society of Medical Oncology; 2004.

[50] Rankin C, von Mehren M, Blanke C, et al. Dose effect of imatinib (IM) in patients (pts) with metastatic GIST—Phase III Sarcoma Group Study S0033. Proc Am Soc Clin Oncol 2004; 22:9005a.

[51] Blay J, Berthaud P, Perol D, et al. Continuous vs intermittent imatinib treatment in advanced GIST after one year: a prospective randomized phase III trial of the French Sarcoma Group. Proc Am Soc Clin Oncol 2004;22:9006a.

[52] Mol CD, Dougan DR, Schneider TR, et al. Structural basis for the autoinhibition and STI-571 inhibition of c-Kit tyrosine kinase. J Biol Chem 2004;279:31655–63.

[53] Lasota J, Jasinski M, Sarlomo-Rikala M, et al. Mutations in exon 11 of c-Kit occur preferentially in malignant versus benign gastrointestinal stromal tumors and do not occur in leiomyomas or leiomyosarcomas. Am J Pathol 1999;154(1):53–60.

[54] Lasota J, Wozniak A, Sarlomo-Rikala M, et al. Mutations in exons 9 and 13 of KIT gene are rare events in gastrointestinal stromal tumors. A study of 200 cases. Am J Pathol 2000;157(4): 1091–5.

[55] Rubin B, Singer S, Tsao C, et al. Activation is a ubiquitous feature of gastrointestinal stromal tumors. Cancer Res 2001;61:8118–21.

[56] Heinrich M, Corless C, Blanke C, et al. KIT mutational status predicts response to STI571 in patients with metastatic gastrointestinal tumors (GISTs). Proc Am Soc Clin Oncol 2002;21:6a.

[57] Heinrich M, Corless C, Demetri G, et al. Kinase mutations and imatinib mesylate response in patients with metastatic gastrointestinal stromal tumor. J Clin Oncol 2003;21:4342–9.

[58] Demetri G, Rankin C, Fletcher C, et al. Phase III dose-randomized study of imatinib mesylate (Gleevec, sti571) for GIST: Intergroup S0033 early results. Proc Am Soc Clin Oncol 2002; 21:1651a.

[59] Tamborini E, Bonadiman L, Greco A, et al. A new mutation in the KIT ATP pocket causes acquired resistance to imatinib in a gastrointestinal stromal tumor patient. Gastroenterology 2004;127:294–9.

[60] Van Oosterom A, Dumez H, Desai J, et al. Combination signal transduction inhibition: a

phase I/II trial of the oral mTOR-inhibitor everolimus (E, RAD001) and imatinib mesylate (IM) in patients (pts) with gastrointestinal stromal tumor (GIST) refractory to IM. Proc Am Soc Clin Oncol 2004;22:3002a.

[61] Reichardt P, Pink P, Lindner T, et al. A phase I/II trial of the oral PKC inhibitor PKC412 and imatinib mesylate in patients with gastrointestinal stromal tumors (GIST) refractory to imatinib (IM). Vienna (Austria): European Society of Medical Oncology; 2004.

[62] Demetri G, George S, Heinrich MC, et al. Clinical activity and tolerability of the multi-targeted tyrosine kinase inhibitor SU11248 in patients (pts) with metastatic gastrointestinal stromal tumor (GIST) refractory to imatinib mesylate [abstract 3273]. Proc Am Soc Clin Oncol 2003;22:814.

[63] Demetri GD, Desai J, Fletcher JA, et al. SU11248, a multi-targeted tyrosine kinase inhibitor, can overcome imatinib (IM) resistance caused by diverse genomic mechanisms in patients (pts) with metastatic gastrointestinal stromal tumor (GIST). Proc Am Soc Clin Oncol 2004;23:3001a.

[64] Heinrich M, Corless C, von Mehren M, et al. PDGFRA and KIT mutations correlate with the clinical responses to imatinib mesylate in patients with advanced gastrointestinal stromal tumors (GIST) [abstract 3274]. Proc Am Soc Clin Oncol 2003;22:815.

[65] Shah N, Tran C, Lee F, et al. Overriding imatinib resistance with a novel ABL kinase inhibitor. Science 2004;305:399–401.

[66] Sawyers C, Shah N, Kantarjian H, et al. Hematologic and cytogenetic responses in imatinib-resistant chronic phase chronic myelogenous leukemia patients treated with the dual SRC/ABL kinase inhibitor BMS-354835: results from a phase I dose escalation study. Blood 2004; 104(11):1a.

[67] Takahashi R, Tanaka S, Kitadai Y, et al. Expression of vascular endothelial growth factor and angiogenesis in gastrointestinal stromal tumor of the stomach. Oncology 2003;64(3):266–74.

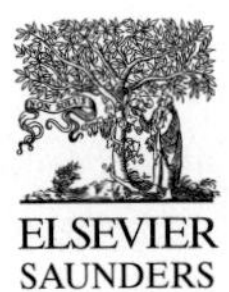

ELSEVIER
SAUNDERS

Hematol Oncol Clin N Am
19 (2005) 565–571

HEMATOLOGY/
ONCOLOGY
CLINICS OF
NORTH AMERICA

Desmoid Tumors and Deep Fibromatoses

Marcus Schlemmer, MD

Medical Clinic and Polyclinic III, Clinic Grosshadern Munich, Ludwig-Maximilian-University Munich, Marchioninistrasse 15, Muenchen D-81377, Germany

The desmoid tumor (also called *deep fibromatosis* or *aggressive fibromatosis*) is a rare, benign tumor entity that was first described in 1832 [1] as a proliferation of fibroblasts. The first report on the association between desmoid tumors and familial adenomatous polyposis (FAP) was published in 1923 [2], and in 1951 Gardner [3] described the simultaneous appearance of intestinal polyposis and fibromas, which is now called "Gardner syndrome." Desmoid tumors are differentiated from more superficial fibromatoses, such as palmar fibromatosis (Dupuytren disease), plantar fibromatosis (Ledderhose disease), penile fibromatosis (Peyronie disease), and knuckle pads, by their location, though these conditions all have a propensity for recurrence and can have trisomy of chromosomes 8 and 14.

Etiology

The etiology of desmoids is poorly understood. Up to 30% of cases have a history including trauma [4,5] and patients who have FAP coli are especially likely to have an occurrence of desmoids after resection of the colon, suggesting genetic influences. Hormones may also play a role in desmoid formation, as abdominal desmoids tend to occur in women during or following pregnancy.

Given their association with FAP, links to the Wnt/beta-catenin pathway have been identified. FAP associated and spontaneous desmoid tumors express beta-

E-mail address: Marcus.Schlemmer@med.uni-muenchen.de

doi:10.1016/j.hoc.2005.03.008

catenin, and even spontaneous desmoids will contain adenomatous polyposis coli (APC) or beta-catenin mutations [6], identifying an important pathway that may provide opportunities for therapy. Furthermore, stabilization of beta-catenin is sufficient to reproduce desmoids in a model system [7]. Like Wilms' tumor, in which WT1 is overexpressed and has beta-catenin mutations, WT1 is also overexpressed in desmoid tumors, pointing out another pathway of potential etiological and therapeutic relevance in this condition [8].

Clinical presentation

Desmoid tumors derive from connective tissue of muscles, the fascia, or the aponeurosis and occur at multiple anatomic sites. Principal sites of involvement are head and neck, shoulder, back, chest wall, abdomen, and thigh (Fig. 1). The most common extra-abdominal sites are shoulder, chest wall, and inguinal region [9], although 30% to 50% of desmoids arise in the abdominal cavity [10,11]. Desmoids are more common among women than men and may occur at any age. The lesions are bulky and show an infiltrative pattern of growth and a tendency to reoccur, though they do not metastasize. Desmoids occur in 12% of patients who have familial adenomatous polyposis [12].

Histology

Microscopically, desmoids present with bundles of spindle cells in a collagenous stroma (Fig. 2). The fibroblasts concentrate at the periphery of the lesion and the cellularity is low. Characteristic criteria of malignancy,

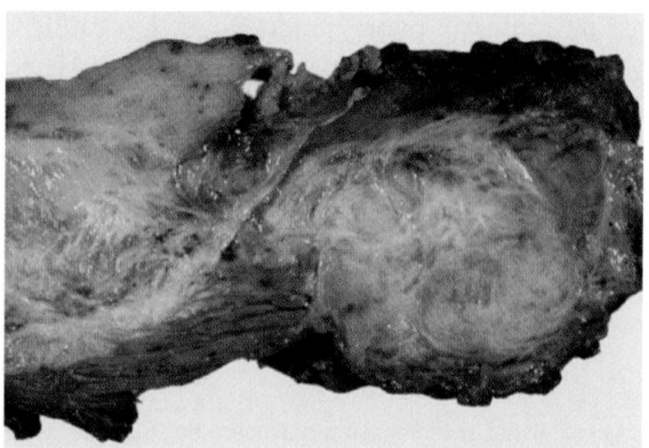

Fig. 1. Aggressive fibromatosis of the thigh. (Courtesy of Professor J. Diebold, Pathology Department, University Grosshadern, Munich, Germany.)

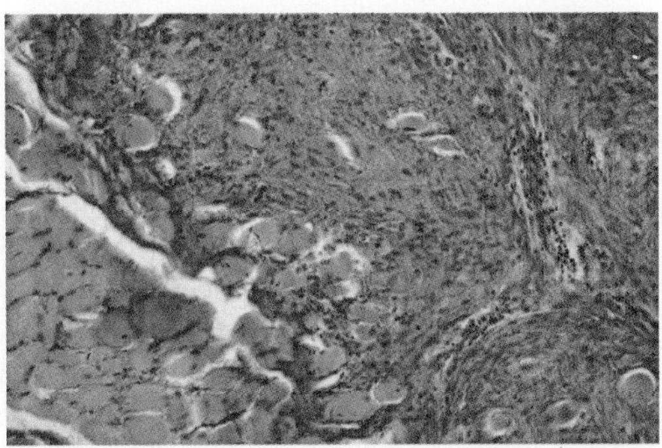

Fig. 2. Histology of the aggressive fibromatosis of the thigh (pictured in Fig. 1). (Courtesy of Professor J. Diebold, Pathology Department, University Grosshadern, Munich, Germany.)

such as mitotic figures or nuclear pleomorphism, are rare [13]. Desmoids lack pseudoencapsulation.

Genetics

Approximately 30% of desmoids show numerical chromosomal aberrations of chromosome 8 (trisomy 8) or chromosome 20 (trisomy 20), but currently there is no clinical relevancy. Data suggest that trisomy may predict recurrence [14]. Inactivation of the APC protein on chromosome 5 (5q) is found in patients who have familial polyposis [15], with most desmoids harboring beta-catenin activating mutations [6].

Diagnosis

Ultrasound is the recommended method for the first differential diagnosis of a soft tissue lesion. To determine adherence to organ structures and respectability, contrast CT scans or MRI are needed. Prediction of resectability concerning margins is only possible with contrast enhanced MRI, but infiltrative growth can often not be assessed sufficiently. As it is not possible to distinguish desmoids from sarcomas by imaging, histologic diagnosis is mandatory. For follow-ups to detect recurrence, ultrasound is feasible and cost-effective.

Treatment

Treatment usually begins with surgical excision of the desmoid tumor. The surgical strategy for desmoid tumors is to obtain tumor-free margins of 1 to 5 cm using function-preserving approaches and avoiding mutilation. The literature presents conflicting data concerning the importance of complete resection. Some authors report recurrence independent of negative margins [16–19], whereas others demonstrate higher local recurrence rate after close or positive margins and postulate aggressive resection [20]. A retrospective analysis of 189 patients treated at M. D. Anderson Cancer Center revealed that the microscopic surgical margin was the single most significant determinant of recurrence in patients treated with surgery [21]. If free margins are not achievable because of adjacent vascular or nerve structures, a distance of less than 1 cm is accepted. In this case radiotherapy should be considered, and can offset the presence of positive margins. It should be noted that a positive margin did not condemn patients to local recurrence. Of 40 patients who had positive margins in the M. D. Anderson Cancer Center study, the 10-year relapse rate was 54% [21].

Ewing [22] mentioned the radioresponsiveness of fibromatoses as "slow but satisfactory" in 1928 and today there is still controversy concerning the role of radiotherapy in the treatment of desmoids. In patients who had initially inoperable lesions, the primary radiation showed that recurrence could be prevented if a median dose of 55 Gy was applied [21,23,24]. The retrospective analysis of 72 patients at the University of Florida, with more than the half of the patients being radiated because of disease recurrence, achieved a locoregional control rate of 83%. Most of the failures in this analysis occurred in the margins of the irradiation field despite careful physical and radiographic evaluation [25]. Because of infiltrative growth of these tumors, margins are often underestimated. Chew et al [26] analyzed patients who had extremity desmoids with median follow-up of 12.5 years and found that the relapse rate after surgery and radiotherapy was 62% after treatment for primary disease. In this analysis, radiation therapy did not reduce relapse rate but prolonged the time to recurrence. A review of published articles on surgery and radiation or both on aggressive fibromatoses by Nuyttens et al [27] revealed a local control rate of 61% for surgery alone, 75% for the combination therapy, and 78% for radiation alone. The American College of Surgeons Oncology group and the European Organization for Research and Treatment of Cancer Soft Tissue Sarcoma Group performed a randomized phase 3 trial to answer the question of adjuvant radiotherapy in aggressive fibromatosis. Despite surgery and radiation therapy, up to 35% of patients show recurrence of their disease [28,29]. Patients who do not have good options for surgery or radiation can be treated pharmacologically.

Systemic therapy for desmoid tumors

Clinical and experimental evidence suggest a role of hormonal dependency in desmoid growth. Cytosolic estrogen receptors and antiestrogen binding sites have been detected in biopsy specimen of desmoid tumors [30]. However, consistent expression is not observed in all patients. Antiestrogen therapy with tamoxifen has shown significant tumor regression in some patients [31,32], but these are often case reports. Therefore, no firm conclusion on tamoxifen effectiveness in desmoids can be drawn. Other hormonal agents have been tested, of which toremifene was effective in first- and second-line treatment [33].

The combination of antiinflammatory agents with antiestrogens demonstrated response rates up to 70% [31], which led to the practice of using nonsteroidal antiinflammatory drugs (NSAID) alone in the treatment of fibromatoses. One report in the literature shows the resolution of a desmoid tumor being treated with indomethacin and ascorbic acid for 14 months [34].

Investigations on interferon suggest an antiproliferative effect on fibroblasts. Reports in the literature detail the results of therapy with interferon-α or interferon-γ for patients who had no other treatment option, or in the post-resection setting. A general recommendation cannot be drawn from these results because there is no randomized or even phase 2 data describing use of these agents [35–37].

If the combination therapy of noncytotoxic drugs after definite surgery becomes ineffective, combination chemotherapy may be administered in selected cases. First experiences with chemotherapy in aggressive fibromatosis in children were published in 1977 [38]. As the behavior of aggressive fibromatosis was felt comparable to that of sarcomas, single-agent doxorubicin was examined [39] and showed responses for doses between 60 mg/m^2 and 90 mg/m^2. Doxorubicin was never tested in a single-agent chemotherapy trial, and because of cardiotoxicity, should not be administered without a cardiac protectant in lifetime cumulative doses more than 300 mg/m^2, according to the American Society of Clinical Oncology guidelines. The combination of vinblastine and methotrexate is effective in children and adults [40–42] and less toxic than the vincristine-dactinomycin-cyclophosphamide regime, although a combination of vinorelbine and methotrexate may be more tolerable compared with vinblastine and vinorelbine [43]. As desmoids express c-kit and appear to express platelet-derived growth factor receptor-α, treatment with the tyrosine-kinase inhibitor imatinib may be beneficial for patients progressing under other therapeutic options [41,44], but remains the subject of clinical investigation.

Summary

Treatment of aggressive fibromatosis remains a clinical challenge. Although desmoids are a benign tumor entity, their locally aggressive behavior and tendency to relapse require multimodality in treatment, consisting of surgery, radiation, and pharmacologic treatment by a team specialized in sarcoma treatment. Even if the gold standard is the primary resection, there are data supporting a “wait and see” strategy in stable, asymptomatic desmoids. Radiation alone in gross tumors can achieve comparable results to surgery. The aggressiveness of the tumor should be matched to the aggressiveness of the therapy. For slowly changing desmoids, noncytotoxic therapy with NSAIDs should be the first step in pharmacologic treatment (keeping in mind newly recognized cardiac risks of NSAIDs), followed by tamoxifen if there is progression. Interferon has potential, but too little data are available for this to be a viable treatment option. If the disease continues to progresses, chemotherapy should be administered. Response rates up to 50% are reportedly achievable with a combination of methotrexate and vinblastine; a combination of vincristin, dactinomycin, and cyclophosphamide; or doxorubicin alone. An international, multicenter trial is essential to establish a standard therapy for patients who have aggressive fibromatosis.

References

[1] MacFarlane J. Clinical reports on the surgical practise of Glasgow Royal Infirmary. Glasgow (Scotland): D. Robertson; 1832. p. 63–7.
[2] Nichols RW. Desmoid tumors: a report of 31 cases. Arch Surg 1923;7:227–36.
[3] Gardner EJ. A genetic and clinical study of intestinal polyposis, a predisposing factor for carcinoma of the colon and rectum. Am J Hum Genet 1951;3:167–76.
[4] Lopez R, Kemalyan N, Moseley HS, et al. Problems in diagnosis and management of desmoid tumors. Am J Surg 1990;159:450–3.
[5] McKinnon JG, Neifeld JP, Kay S, et al. Management of desmoid tumors. Surg Gynecol Obstet 1989;169:104–6.
[6] Tejpar S, Nollet F, Li C, et al. Predominance of beta-catenin mutations and beta-catenin dysregulation in sporadic aggressive fibromatosis (desmoid tumor). Oncogene 1999;18:6615–20.
[7] Cheon SS, Cheah AY, Turley S, et al. Beta-catenin stabilization dysregulates mesenchymal cell proliferation, motility, and invasiveness and causes aggressive fibromatosis and hyperplastic cutaneous wounds. Proc Natl Acad Sci USA 2002;99:6973–8.
[8] Amini Nik S, Hohenstein P, Jadidzadeh A, et al. Upregulation of Wilms' tumor gene 1 (WT1) in desmoid tumors. Int J Cancer 2005;114:202–8.
[9] Khorsand J, Karakousis CP. Desmoid tumours and their management. Am J Surg 1985;149: 215–8.
[10] Reitamo JJ, Häyry P, Nykyri E, et al. The desmoid tumor. I. Incidence, sex, age and anatomical distribution in the Finnish population. Am J Clin Pathol 1982;77:665–73.
[11] Burke AP, Sobin LH, Shekitka KM, et al. Intra-abdominal fibromatosis: a pathologic analysis of 130 tumors with comparison of clinical subgroups. Am J Surg Pathol 1990;14:335–41.
[12] Church JM, McGannon E. Prior pregnancy ameliorates the course of intra-abdominal desmoid tumors in patients with familial adenomatous polyposis. Dis Colon Rectum 2000;43: 445–50.
[13] Enzinger FM, Weiss SW. Soft tissue tumors. 3rd edition. St. Louis (MO): Mosby; 1995. p. 201–29.
[14] Fletcher JA, Naeem R, Xiao S, et al. Chromosome aberrations in desmoid tumours: trisomy 8 may be a predictor of recurrence. Cancer Genet Cytogenet 1995;63:527–9.
[15] Leppert M, Dobbs M, Scrambler P, et al. The gene for familial polyposis maps to the long arm of chromosome 5. Science 1987;238:1411–3.
[16] Kiel KD, Suit HD. Radiation therapy in the treatment of aggressive fibromatoses (desmoid tumors). Cancer 1984;54:2051–4.
[17] Reitamo JJ. The desmoid tumor. IV: Choice of treatment, results and complications. Arch Surg 1983;118:1318–22.
[18] Mirabell R, Suit HD, Mankin HJ, et al. Fibromatoses: from postsurgical surveillance to combined surgery and radiation therapy. Int J Radiat Oncol Biol Phys 1990;18:535–54.
[19] Gronchi A, Casali PG, Mariani L, et al. Quality of surgery and outcome in extra-abdominal aggressive fibromatosis: a series of patients surgically treated at a single institution. J Clin Oncol 2003;21:1390–7.

[20] Posner MC, Shiu MH, Newsome JL, et al. The desmoid tumor. Not a benign disease. Arch Surg 1989;124:191–6.
[21] Ballo MT, Zagars GK, Pollack A, et al. Desmoid tumor: prognostic factors and outcome after surgery, radiation therapy, or combined surgery and radiation therapy. J Clin Oncol 1999;17: 158–67.
[22] Ewing J. Neoplastic diseases. 2nd edition. Philadelphia: WB Saunders; 1928.
[23] Spear MA, Jennings LC, Mankin HJ, et al. Individualizing management of aggressive fibromatosis. Int J Radiat Oncol Biol Phys 1998;40:637–45.
[24] Bataini JP, Belloir C, Mazarbraud A, et al. Desmoid tumors in adults: the role of radiotherapy in their management. Am J Surg 1988;155:754–60.
[25] Zlotecki RA, Scarborough MT, Morris CG, et al. External beam radiotherapy for primary and adjuvant management of aggressive fibromatosis. Int J Radiat Oncol Biol Phys 2002;54:177–81.
[26] Chew C, Reid R, O'Dwyer PJ. Evaluation of the long term outcome of patients with extremity desmoids. Eur J Surg Oncol 2004;30:428–32.
[27] Nuyttens JJ, Rust PF, Thomas Jr CR, et al. Surgery versus radiation therapy for patients with aggressive fibromatosis or desmoid tumors. Cancer 2000;88:1517–23.
[28] Pritchard DJ, Nascimento AG, Petersen IA, et al. Local control of extraabdominal desmoid tumors. J Bone Joint Surg 1996;78:848–54.
[29] Sherman NE, Romsdahl M, Evans H, et al. Desmoid tumors: a 20-year radiotherapy experience. Int J Radiat Oncol Biol Phys 1990;19:37–40.
[30] Lim CL, Walker MJ, Mehta RR, et al. Estrogen and antiestrogen binding sites in desmoid tumors. Eur J Cancer Clin Oncol 1986;22:583–7.
[31] Hansmann A, Adolph C, Vogel T, et al. High-dose tamoxifen and sulindac as first-line treatment for desmoid tumors. Cancer 2004;100:612–20.
[32] Lackner H, Urban C, Benesch M, et al. Multimodal treatment of children with unresectable or recurrent desmoid tumors: an 11-year longitudinal observational study. J Pediatr Hematol Oncol 2004;26:518–22.
[33] Brooks MD, Ebbs SR, Coletta AA, et al. Desmoid tumors treated with triphenylethylenes. Eur J Cancer 1992;28A:1014–8.
[34] Waddell WR, Garner RE. Indomethacin and ascorbate inhibit desmoid tumors. J Surg Oncol 1980;15:85–90.
[35] Acker JC, Bossen EH, Halperin EC. The management of desmoid tumours. Int J Radiat Oncol Phys 1993;26:851–8.
[36] Leithner A, Schnack B, Katterschafka T, et al. Treatment of extraabdominal desmoid tumors with interferon-alpha with or without tretinoin. J Surg Oncol 2000;73:21–5.
[37] Raguse JD, Gath HJ, Oettle H, et al. Interferon-induced remission of rapidly growing aggressive fibromatosis in the temporal fossa. Int J Oral Maxillofac Surg 2004;33:606–9.
[38] Stein R. Chemotherapeutic response in fibromatosis of the neck. J Pediatr 1977;90:482–3.
[39] Seiter K, Kemeny N. Successful treatment of a desmoid tumor with doxorubicin. Cancer 1993; 71:2242–4.
[40] Okuno SH, Edmonson JH. Combination chemotherapy for desmoid tumors. Cancer 2003;97: 1134–5.
[41] Skapec SX, Hawk BJ, Hoffer FA, et al. Combination chemotherapy using vinblastine and methotrexate for the treatment of progressive desmoid tumor in children. J Clin Oncol 1998; 16:3021–7.
[42] Azzarelli A, Gronchi A, Bertulli R, et al. Low-dose chemotherapy with methotrexate and vinblastine for patients with advanced aggresive fibromatosis. Cancer 2001;92(5):1259–64.
[43] Weiss AJ, Horowitz S, Lackman RD. Therapy of desmoid tumors and fibromatosis using vinorelbine. Am J Clin Oncol 1999;22:193–5.
[44] Mace J, Biermann JS, Sondak V, et al. Response of extraabdominal desmoid tumors to therapy with imatinib mesylate. Cancer 2002;95:2373–9.

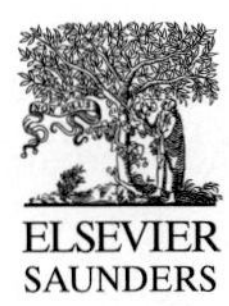
ELSEVIER
SAUNDERS

Hematol Oncol Clin N Am
19 (2005) 573–590

HEMATOLOGY/
ONCOLOGY
CLINICS OF
NORTH AMERICA

Recent Studies in Novel Therapy for Metastatic Sarcomas

Dejka M. Steinert, MD[a], Shreyaskumar R. Patel, MD[b,*]

[a]*Division of Cancer Medicine, The University of Texas, MD Anderson Cancer Center, Unit 10, 1515 Holcombe Boulevard, Houston, TX 77030, USA*

[b]*Department of Sarcoma Medical Oncology, The University of Texas, MD Anderson Cancer Center, Unit 450, 1515 Holcombe Boulevard, Houston, TX 77030, USA*

Gemcitabine and combinations

Several groups have studied the nucleoside analog gemcitabine in soft tissue sarcoma (STS) with variable results depending on study design and patient population. We performed a two-arm phase 2 study of the nucleoside analog gemcitabine in patients who had advanced soft-tissue sarcomas. We studied the weekly schedule of the drug at a dose of 1000 mg/m^2 every week for up to 7 weeks followed by a 1-week break and restaging. Responding patients subsequently continued with the same weekly dose for 3 weeks followed by a 1-week break. One arm included patients previously treated for soft-tissue sarcoma, excluding those who had gastrointestinal stromal tumors (GISTs), in whom we saw seven partial responses (PR) out of 39 patients for a response rate of 18% (95% CI, 7%–29%). The median duration of response was 3.5 months, with a range from 2 to 13 months. Four of the ten patients who had leiomyosarcoma of nongastrointestinal origin achieved a PR, suggesting the possibility of some selective activity in this subset. In the other arm, comprised of patients who had GISTs, no objective responses were achieved in 17 evaluable patients, and that arm was therefore discontinued. Comparison of cellular pharmacology demonstrated a 1.4-fold increase in the concentration of gem-

* Corresponding author.
E-mail address: spatel@mdanderson.org (S.R. Patel).

0889-8588/05/$ – see front matter
doi:10.1016/j.hoc.2005.03.002

citabine triphosphate with more prolonged (150-minute) infusion. The median survival for the entire study population was 13.9 months [1].

Investigators from Memorial Sloan Kettering Cancer Center conducted a phase 2 trial of gemcitabine and docetaxel in patients who had unresectable leiomyosarcoma [2]. Participants in this trial included 29 patients who had unresectable uterine leiomyosarcoma and five patients who had unresectable leiomyosarcoma of other primary sites who had been treated with no prior chemotherapy or up to two prior regimens. Patients received gemcitabine 900 mg/m^2 intravenously on days 1 and 8 plus docetaxel 100 mg/m^2 on day 8 with granulocyte colony-stimulating factor given subcutaneously on days 9 to 15, with cycles repeated every 21 days. For those patients who had received prior pelvic radiation, the dose of both chemotherapy agents was decreased by 25%. Gemcitabine was infused over 30 or 90 minutes for cycles one and two and over 90 minutes for all subsequent cycles. Of the 34 patients enrolled on this trial, 14 had received prior pelvic radiation, 16 had progressed after doxorubicin-based therapy, and 18 had no prior chemotherapy. The overall response rate was 53% (95% CI, 35%–70%), with three complete responses and 15 partial responses. Half of the patients previously treated with doxorubicin responded. This regimen was well tolerated with manageable hematologic toxicity (neutropenia: grade 3, 15%; grade 4, 6%; thrombocytopenia: grade 3, 26%; grade 4, 3%) and rare neutropenic fever (6%). The median time to progression was 5.6 months [2]. This study demonstrates that gemcitabine combined with docetaxel is well tolerated and highly active in untreated and previously treated patients who have leiomyosarcoma, especially of uterine origin.

Hensley and colleagues [3] expanded the above phase 2 trial to include patients who had histologies other than leiomyosarcoma and gave an update of the longer-term progression-free and overall survival for those patients who had leiomyosarcoma. The expanded phase 2 trial spanned from June 1999 through April 2003 and included a total of 52 patients, of whom 42 had leiomyosarcoma and 10 had some other type of sarcoma. The dose and schedule of gemcitabine and docetaxel was the same for the expanded trial compared with the original trial design. Patients could receive up to a maximum of eight on-study cycles of this chemotherapy. The overall response rate was 35% (95% CI, 22%–48%). The response rate was significantly better in those patients who had leiomyosarcoma compared with nonleiomyosarcoma histologies (40% versus 10%, respectively). Only 15% of patients had grade 3 to 4 toxicities, consisting mostly of myelosuppression. For patients who had leiomyosarcoma, progression-free survival at 6 months was 35% (95% CI, 20%–49%) and overall survival at 2 years was 47% (95% CI, 31%–63%). For the 18 patients who had an objective response, the median duration of response was 7 months [3]. This expanded trial confirmed that the combination of gemcitabine and docetaxel is an active regimen for patients who have leiomyosarcoma. No definitive conclusions can be drawn from this trial regarding the use of this combination in other STSs secondary to the small sample size of patients who have nonleiomyosarcoma histologies. Hopefully, the current ongoing multicenter study that is looking at gemcitabine versus gemcitabine combined with docetaxel in patients who have metastatic STS will provide additional information.

Another phase 2 trial looked at the use of gemcitabine in uterine leiomyosarcoma, but this time as a single agent in those patients who had recurrent or persistent uterine leiomyosarcoma [4]. The dosing schedule was slightly different in this, trial with 1000 mg/m^2 gemcitabine given intravenously over 30 minutes on days 1, 8, and 15 every 28 days. Although 48 patients were enrolled in this trial, only 44 were evaluable for toxicity and 42 for toxicity and response; 35 patients had previously received chemotherapy and 11 patients had prior radiotherapy. This regimen was well tolerated with the only grade 4 toxicities consisting of neutropenia (n = 7), nausea and vomiting (n = 2), and skin (n = 1). The overall response rate was 20.5% with one (2.3%) complete response and eight (18.2%) partial responses [4].

Gemcitabine in combination with vinorelbine has been evaluated in a single institution phase 2 study as a first- or second-line chemotherapy regimen for patients who have metastatic STS [5]. Gemcitabine was given at 800 mg/m^2 infused over 90 minutes on days 1 and 8 of a 21-day cycle, following vinorelbine at a dose of 25 mg/m^2. Of the 18 patients enrolled in this trial, nine had uterine or extremity leiomyosarcoma, two had high-grade pleomorphic sarcoma, and one each had carcinosarcoma, pleomorphic liposarcoma, malignant peripheral nerve sheath tumor, desmoplastic small round cell tumor, rhabdomyosarcoma, and small round cell tumor. The most common grade 3 and 4 toxicities were hematologic, with all three grade 4 toxicities and 10 out of 19 grade 3 toxicities being hematologic. Three patients benefited from this regimen with either a partial response or stable disease for more than 4 months. The patients benefiting consisted of one patient who had high-grade uterine leiomyosarcoma who achieved a PR, one patient who had a small round cell tumor who achieved a PR, and one patient who had metastatic malignant peripheral nerve sheath tumor who had stable disease. Thus far, median time to progression has been 4.2 months and median survival 6.25 [5]. Further accrual to this study and a longer follow-up is necessary to determine if the combination of gemcitabine and vinorelbine will play a role in the treatment of metastatic STSs in the future.

Imatinib mesylate in gastrointestinal stromal tumors

Phase 1 trials

The initial phase 1 studies of imatinib mesylate were conducted in patients who had chronic myeloid leukemia (CML). The first phase 1 trial of imatinib mesylate was performed between June 1998 and May 2000 at three participating study centers [6]. Eighty-three patients who had CML in the chronic phase in whom treatment with interferon had failed were successively assigned to one of 14 doses ranging from 25 to 1000 mg/d. The primary endpoint of this dose escalation study was the safety and tolerability of imatinib mesylate in patients who had chronic-phase CML. Doses of this drug were administered orally once daily, except for the 800- and 1000-mg doses, which were divided into two daily doses. Toxicity was minimal in this study and included nausea, myalgias, edema, and diarrhea. A maximal tolerated dose was not defined, and imatinib mesylate was found to have significant antileukemic activity [6].

A single-patient pilot study confirmed the efficacy of imatinib mesylate in GIST [7]. This first patient to be treated with imatinib mesylate was a 50-year-old woman who had chemotherapy-resistant, metastatic GIST who received once-daily doses of 400 mg of imatinib mesylate starting in March 2000. This patient's tumor had previously been documented to express the Kit receptor (CD117) and was subsequently found to encode a mutation in exon 11 of the *kit* gene. Response was evaluated objectively, using 18-fluorodeoxyglucose (FDG) positron emission tomography (PET) and CT radiography. The patient's tumor remained stable after a year of therapy, and she had only mild gastrointestinal adverse effects. Serial tumor biopsies revealed myxoid degeneration after only 4 weeks of treatment [7].

A phase 1 study of imatinib mesylate in GIST was done in three centers of the European Organization for Research and Treatment of Cancer (EORTC) Soft Tissue and Bone Sarcoma Group [8]. The goal of this trial was to identify the dose-limiting adverse effects of imatinib mesylate in patients who have metastatic GIST. Initially, this trial was designed for patients who had any advanced STS, including GIST, but ultimately, 36 of the 40 patients enrolled had advanced GIST. Between August 3, 2000, and December 21, 2000, the patients received imatinib mesylate at doses of 400 mg once daily, 300 mg twice daily, 400 mg twice daily, or 500 mg twice daily. The maximum tolerated dose of imatinib mesylate was judged to be 400 mg twice daily, owing to unacceptable toxicity at the 500 mg twice daily dose, which included grade 3 nausea/vomiting, edema, and dyspnea. Although not the primary endpoint, a partial response rate of 69% was reported [8].

Phase 2 trials

These encouraging results and the experience of using imatinib mesylate in patients who had CML led to the rapid deployment of several phase 2 and phase 3 studies of imatinib mesylate in GIST. The initial trial, designated as the US-Finland trial [9] was a multicenter, open-label, randomized phase 2 clinical trial of imatinib mesylate in patients who had unresectable or metastatic, Kit-expressing GIST. Between July 2000 and April 2001, 147 patients were randomly assigned to receive 400 or 600 mg of imatinib mesylate daily through oral administration. This study had a crossover design: patients receiving 400 mg daily whose tumors progressed but who were otherwise in good clinical condition were eligible to increase the dose to 600 mg daily. After a median follow-up of 41 weeks, imatinib mesylate was shown to be effective and to have minimal toxicity, with 54% of patients having a partial response and another 28% demonstrating stable disease. Although there were no complete responses, only

14% of patients exhibited disease progression. Equivalent response rates were seen in the two treatment arms, but this phase 2 study was not adequately powered to distinguish a difference in efficacy between the 400-mg and 600-mg doses [9].

At a median follow-up of 24 months, 63% of patients in the US-Finland trial had a partial response, 19% of patients had stable disease, and 12% had confirmed tumor progression [10]. The median time to progression was 72 weeks, and the median survival had yet to be reached. The response rates did not differ significantly between the two doses, although there was a trend toward a higher response rate at the 600-mg dose (65% versus 62%) [10].

The above results were confirmed with another phase 2 trial performed by the EORTC Soft Tissue and Bone Sarcoma Group [11]. The goal of this study was to assess the activity of imatinib mesylate in advanced or metastatic GIST at the highest feasible dose of 400 mg twice daily. A total of 27 patients who had GIST were enrolled on this trial. Adverse effects were mild to moderate, and the most common included anemia, periorbital edema, skin rash, fatigue, nausea, granulocytopenia, and diarrhea. Response rates were similar to those in the US-Finland phase 2 trial: 4% complete response, 67% partial response, 18% stable disease, and 11% disease progression. At 1 year, 73% of patients were free from disease progression [11].

Phase 3 trials

Two phase 3 studies were conducted nearly simultaneously by two large consortia. One was the North American Sarcoma Intergroup study S0033, consisting of the United States cooperative oncology groups (Southwest Oncology Group, Cancer and Leukemia Group B, and the Eastern Cooperative Group) and the National Cancer Institute of Canada Sarcoma Group [12,13]. The primary aim of this study was to assess the impact of imatinib mesylate dose (400 mg versus 800 mg daily) on survival; secondary aims were to evaluate response rates and confirm the tolerability of imatinib mesylate therapy in patients who have GIST. Between December 15, 2000, and September 1, 2001, 746 patients from 57 institutions were enrolled. Patients randomized to receive the 400 mg daily dose were allowed to cross over to the 800 mg daily dose if they had radiographic evidence of progressive disease. Early results of this trial were presented at the American Society of Clinical Oncology (ASCO) annual meeting in 2003 [12]. At a median follow-up of 14 months, overall response rates were similar in both arms: 43% at the 400 mg dose and 41% at the 800 mg dose [12]. There was no difference in progression-free or overall survival between dose levels. The most recent update of this trial was presented at the 2004 ASCO meeting [13]. Median overall survival had not been reached in either arm after a median follow-up of 25.6 months, and there continued to be no significant differences between the two arms regarding progression-free and overall survival. Progression-free survival rate estimates at 2 years are 50% versus 53% for the 400 mg versus 800 mg arms, respectively. Survival estimates at 2 years are 78% versus 73% for the 400 mg versus 800 mg arms, respectively. However, of the 106 patients who crossed over to the higher dose after having progressive disease on the 400 mg daily dose, 7% had a partial response and 32% had stable disease, indicating that patients can benefit from a higher dose after their disease progresses on 400 mg daily.

The EORTC Soft Tissue and Bone Sarcoma Group, Italian Sarcoma Group, and Australasian Gastro-Intestinal Trials Group conducted the second phase 3 trial of imatinib mesylate [14]. Between February 2001 and February 2002, 946 patients who had GIST were randomized to receive imatinib mesylate at a dose of either 400 mg daily or 400 mg twice daily. This trial was powered to detect a 10% difference in progression-free survival rates, with objective response to treatment as a secondary endpoint. At a median follow-up of 760 days (approximately 25 months), 56% of patients on the once-daily arm had progressed compared with only 50% of patients on the twice-a-day arm (estimated hazard ratio 0.82 [95% CI, 0.69–0.98]; $P = .026$). The benefit in terms of median progression-free survival was an extra 5 months for those patients on the 400 mg twice-a-day arm. Fifty-two (5%) patients achieved a complete response, 442 (47%) patients achieved a partial response, and 300 (32%) patients had stable disease. The median time to best response was 107 days. The significance of this trial is that although both arms achieved the same induction response, the dose of 400 mg twice a day achieved a significantly longer progression-free survival. Overall survival estimates at 1 year are 85% and 86% for the once-daily and twice-daily arms, respectively. At 2 years, overall survival estimates are 69% and 74% for the once-daily and twice-daily arms, respectively [14]. The North American trial did not show a statistically significant difference in progression-free survival, and the reason for this discrepancy is unknown, although differences in site of *kit* mutation, differences in racial composition between the two studies, and the larger size of the EORTC study could be considered.

Safety and tolerability of imatinib

The US-Finland phase 2 trial demonstrated that imatinib mesylate was generally well tolerated [9]. However, virtually every patient had at least some mild or moderate adverse events (grade 1 or 2) that were attributable to therapy [9]. The most common adverse events were edema (which was most frequently periorbital), nausea, diarrhea, myalgia or musculoskeletal pain, fatigue, rash, headache, and abdominal pain. Although most of these adverse events were mild or moderate, 21% of patients experienced serious adverse events (grade 3 or 4). A few patients (5%) experienced intraabdominal hemorrhages [9], which were postulated to be associated with massive tumor cell death induced by this active agent.

The most recent toxicity results of the large phase 3 trial conducted by the EORTC Soft Tissue and Bone Sarcoma Group, Italian Sarcoma Group, and Australasian Gastro-Intestinal Trials Group were reported at a median follow-up of 760 days (approximately 25 months) [14]. Almost all patients in both arms (400 mg of imatinib daily versus twice daily) had some type of adverse effect: 468 out of 472 (99%) in the twice-daily arm and 465 out of 470 (99%) in the once-daily arm. The most common hematologic events were anemia (879 patients, 93%) and granulocytopenia (395, 42%). Hemoglobin levels fell by a median of 8% compared with initial values in patients taking 400 mg daily and by a median of 13% in patients taking 800 mg daily. The most common nonhematologic adverse effects were edema (748, 80%), fatigue (693, 74%), nausea (515, 55%), pleuritic pain (500, 53%), diarrhea (494, 52%), and rash (345, 37%). Patients taking the higher dose of imatinib were more likely to have at least one grade 3 to 4 adverse effect (152 [32%] on once-daily treatment compared with 237 [50%] on twice-daily treatment; $P < .001$). Also, patients on the twice-a-day arm were more likely to have certain adverse effects (edema, anemia, rash, lethargy, nausea, bleeding, diarrhea, and dyspnea) compared with those patients on the once-a-day arm. However, serious adverse events were reported equally for both arms: 174 (37%) for the once-daily arm versus 180 (38%) for the twice-daily arm. Imatinib was the most probable cause of death in five (0.5%) patients (two patients on the once-a-day arm, and three on the twice-a-day arm). In an additional 13 (1%) patients, imatinib could not be completely ruled out as the cause of death. Hepatic toxic events (three patients) and bleeding (two patients) were thought to be the cause of death in five patients.

Dose reductions were much more likely in patients taking imatinib 400 mg twice a day compared with those on the once-a-day arm (282 [60%] versus 77 [16%], $P < .001$). The reason for a dose reduction was more likely to be a nonhematologic rather than a hematologic toxic effect in either arm. Patients on the higher dose of imatinib were more likely to need a treatment interruption (302 [64%] versus 189 [40%], $P < .001$), most often from a nonhematologic rather than a hematologic toxic effect. In summary, imatinib mesylate is safe and generally well tolerated at doses up to 800 mg daily.

SU11248

An increasing number of patients who have GIST are becoming resistant to imatinib and are in need of other treatment options. Imatinib resistance has been correlated with the appearance of secondary mutations in the Kit or platelet-derived growth factor receptor α (PDGFRA) tyrosine kinases in GIST lesions refractory to imatinib [14a]. Activation of alternative signaling pathways and a different structural biology of the new mutant kinases contribute to the growing problem of the emergence of imatinib-resistant GIST clones. SU11248 is an oral drug that inhibits specific tyrosine kinases: vascular endothelial growth factor (VEGF), platelet-derived growth factor (PDGF), Kit, and Flt 2. A phase 1/2 clinical trial of SU11248 is currently underway in patients who have progressing imatinib-resistant GISTs [15]. In this trial, investigators obtained tumor biopsies to define the mutational status of the Kit and PDGFRA kinases by denaturing high pressure liquid chromatography and sequencing assays. Thus far, 98 patients who have progressive GIST have been enrolled, with tumor response data available in 48 patients and GIST genotype determined in 41. Patients received SU11248 at an oral dose of 50 mg daily for 4 weeks followed by a 2-week period off of the drug in each 6-week cycle. In the 48 evaluable patients, 26 (54%) had a clinical benefit, defined as an objective response or stable disease for 6 months. Six (13%) out of the 48 patients had a confirmed partial response. In this trial, Kit exon 11 mutants had more secondary mutations than Kit exon 9 GISTs. Those patients who had Kit exon 9 mutants were more likely to have clinical benefit (PR and stable disease >6 months) to SU11248 than those who had Kit exon 11 mutants: 11 out of 14 (79%) versus 8 out of 24 (33%), respectively. Because patients who have GIST resistant to imatinib have been found to respond to SU11248 in the phase 1/2 setting, a phase 3 trial is planned to define further the activity of SU11248 in this patient population [15].

Everolimus

Another agent being evaluated in patients who have GIST refractory or resistant to imatinib is the oral mTOR-inhibitor everolimus (RAD001) [16]. It is believed that resistance to imatinib is possibly caused by other mutations of Kit, genomic amplification of Kit, or activation of alternative oncogenic signaling mechanisms. Studies evaluating the signal-profiling of GIST lesions that initially respond to imatinib and then develop clonal evolution of imatinib-resistant disease demonstrate a close association between Kit and AKT/mTOR activity [16]. With the background knowledge that in vitro data shows synergism between imatinib and everolimus, a phase 1/2 clinical trial has been initiated and is ongoing to test the feasibility of the combination of everolimus and imatinib and to assess the effect of this combination on patients who have GIST refractory to imatinib [16]. The preliminary results of this trial show that in 12 patients, imatinib increases levels of everolimus, but everolimus did not affect the levels of imatinib. Patient tolerance to this combination was good overall. One patient has stable disease after 10 months on study. The investigators in this trial propose that the increase in everolimus bioavailability could be through competition with imatinib for CYP3A4 or P-glycoprotein. This study is ongoing and the investigators are currently testing intercohort dosage escalation of everolimus (2.5–10 mg/d) with imatinib 600 mg daily.

Imatinib mesylate in dermatofibrosarcoma protuberans

Usually dermatofibrosarcoma protuberans (DFSP) is treated with local therapy alone because fewer than 5% of patients develop metastases, but for those patients who develop metastases, prognosis is poor. Imatinib mesylate is a known inhibitor of Abl, Kit, and platelet-derived growth factor beta (PDGFB) tyrosine kinases, whereas DFSP is felt to be caused by activation of PDGFB [17]. For this reason, imatinib mesylate has been tried in metastatic DFSP, and results have been promising. In one case a 25-year-old man who had unresectable, metastatic DFSP was treated with imatinib mesylate 400 mg twice daily for 4 months. Response to treatment was evaluated by FDG PET, MRI, and histopathologic and immunohistochemical evaluation. Within 2 weeks of starting treatment, the hypermetabolic uptake of FDG fell to background levels. After 4 months of therapy, the tumor volume had decreased over 75%, which allowed resection of the mass. Evaluation of the posttreatment tumor mass revealed a complete histologic response with no residual viable tumor identified [18]. This report supported prior suggestions that PDGF receptors could be a target for pharmacologic treatment of DFSP [17]. Two other patients who had metastatic DFSP were treated with imatinib mesylate, 400 mg daily. One of these patients only had a transient response and unfortunately the disease then progressed rapidly and the patient died of disease. The other patient had a partial response after 2 months consisting of resolution of a superior vena cava syndrome and shrinkage of pulmonary metastases. At 6 months, this patient was still receiving treatment and was continuing to respond [19].

More recently reported were the results of ten patients who had DFSP treated with imatinib 800 mg daily [20]. Eight of these patients had locally advanced DFSP and two had metastatic disease. Each of the eight patients who had locally advanced DFSP had karyotypic or fluorescent in situ hybridization evidence of t(17;22), the translocation typically associated with DFSP, and had clinical response to imatinib. Two of these responses were complete clinical responses. The two patients who had metastatic disease had fibrosarcomatous histology, but the karyotypes were substantially more complex than those reported generally in locally advanced DFSP. In one of these patients, the metastatic DFSP had the t(17;22), and this patient initially had a partial response to imatinib but the disease progressed after 7 months of treatment. The other patient who had metastatic disease did not have the t(17;22) and did not respond to imatinib [20]. This study confirms previous findings that imatinib does have clinical activity in localized and metastatic DFSP, especially those that have t(17;22). Whether DFSP tumors that lack t(17;22) will respond to imatinib is yet to be determined.

Imatinib mesylate in desmoid tumors and other sarcomas

Previously, Mace and colleagues [21] demonstrated consistent expression of c-Kit, PDGFR-alpha, and PDGFR-beta in nine desmoid tumors. Two patients whose tumors had been analyzed were then treated with imatinib mesylate at a dosage of 400 mg twice daily. Both of these patients responded to therapy, and the investigators recommended that further study of this drug in patients who have desmoid tumors should be completed in the context of a formal prospective trial [21], currently being conducted by the Sarcoma Alliance for Research through Collaboration (SARC). Thus far, 26 patients who have desmoid tumors who were deemed not be surgical candidates have been enrolled in this trial, and 22 are evaluable. The 2- and 4-month progression-free survival rates for these patients are 91% and 78%, respectively. Polymorphisms/mutations of PDGFR on exon 18 were found on these tumors, and the investigators postulated that responsiveness of desmoid tumors to imatinib mesylate may be a function of alteration of this gene or other downstream effectors [22]. As in dermatofibrosarcoma protuberans, imatinib mesylate shows promise as a systemic therapy for those patients who have desmoid tumors who are not candidates for local therapy alone.

In addition to studying the effectiveness of imatinib mesylate in patients who have unresectable desmoid tumors, the above SARC phase 2 trial is looking at nine other subtypes of sarcoma. The 4-month progression-free survival for three of the subtypes is as follows: liposarcoma 32% (9 out of 28), leiomyosarcoma 20% (6 out of 30), and fibrosarcoma 29% (2 out of 7) [23].

Paclitaxel in angiosarcoma

Paclitaxel in the treatment of advanced or metastatic angiosarcoma shows promise. A phase 2 trial was performed evaluating the effects paclitaxel on 28 participating patients who had soft-tissue sarcomas [24]. Patients who had measurable advanced soft-tissue sarcomas received paclitaxel at 250 mg/m^2 given as a 3-hour intravenous (IV) infusion once every 21 days. Out of the 28 patients, two partial responses (7%; 95% CI, 1%–23%) were observed. One of the responding patients had angiosarcoma of the scalp and pulmonary metastases and had complete regression of cutaneous lesions and improvement of nonmeasurable pulmonary disease that lasted 6 months. The other patient who responded was a woman who had metastatic uterine leiomyosarcoma. Her partial response lasted 9 months. Also, two patients who had angiosarcoma of the scalp who did not qualify for this study were treated with paclitaxel off-protocol and experienced dramatic tumor regression [24].

Based on the encouraging results of their phase 2 trial, the investigators at Memorial Sloan-Kettering Cancer Center reviewed their experience with paclitaxel in the treatment of adult patients who had angiosarcoma of the head and neck [25]. The investigators identified nine patients who had cutaneous angiosarcoma treated with paclitaxel between January 1992 and December 1998. This group of nine patients included the one patient who had angiosarcoma who was enrolled in their phase 2 trial of paclitaxel in STS. The administration of paclitaxel varied with infusions over 1, 3, and 24 hours. Out of these nine patients, eight had major responses (four partial responses and four clinical complete responses), and one patient had a minor response. The major response rate was 89% with a median duration of response of 5 months (range, 2–13 months). Patients tolerated the paclitaxel well with the most frequent dose-limiting toxicities consisting of neutropenia and peripheral neuropathy [25]. Single-agent paclitaxel should be further investigated in patients who have advanced or metastatic angiosarcomas in the setting of a clinical trial to better determine the optimal dose and schedule of paclitaxel.

Paclitaxel and STA-4783

A multi-institution phase 2 study is currently underway looking at the combination of paclitaxel and STA-4783 (SyntaPharma, Lexington, Massachusetts) in patients who have soft-tissue sarcomas not suitable for surgical resection. The precise molecular pathway of STA-4783 is still being delineated, but it is believed that STA-4783 may induce heat shock protein 70 selectively in tumor cells that are undergoing cell death or stress in response to paclitaxel. Patients participating in this trial will receive STA-4783 213 mg/m^2 plus paclitaxel 80 mg/m^2 weekly for 3 weeks, followed by a 1-week rest period. Cycles will be repeated until disease progression. Results of this trial are eagerly anticipated, especially regarding the subset of patients who have angiosarcomas and are treated with this combination.

Ecteinascidin

Ecteinascidin (ET-743; PharmaMar, Madrid, Spain) is a marine-derived compound isolated from the Caribbean marine tunicate *Ecteinascidia turbinate*. The drug covalently binds to the minor groove of the DNA and blocks the cell cycle in late S and G2 phases. It also affects the organization and assembly of the microtubule network. Preliminary evidence of activity was reported in 29 pretreated patients who had advanced bone (n = 4) and soft-tissue sarcomas (n = 25) [26]. Twelve patients were treated in a phase 1 study, and 17 others were treated in a compassionate-use program at doses ranging from 1200 to 1800 μg/m^2. The maximum tolerated dose was 1800 μg/m^2, and the recommended dose was 1500 μg/m^2 as a 24-hour infusion. Two patients who had osteosarcoma and soft-tissue sarcoma achieved a partial response. Two other patients achieved a minor response, and ten patients had stable disease. The median duration of response was 10.5 months (2.8 to 15 months). Toxicities included transient grade 3 and 4 transaminitis in 24% and 5% of the cycles, respectively. Grade 3 and 4 neutropenia and thrombocytopenia occurred in 32% and 5% of cycles, respectively. Twenty-one percent of the cycles were associated with grade 2 and 3 asthenia [26].

Several phase 2 trials have been conducted including a multicenter study, which evaluated efficacy, safety, and pharmacokinetics of ecteinascidin-743 (ET-743) in patients who had pretreated advanced soft-tissue sarcoma [27]. Patients received ET-743 at a dose of 1500 μg/m^2 as a 24-hour IV infusion every 3 weeks. To be eligible for this study, patients were required to have been treated with at least one line of single-agent or combination chemotherapy with progression of disease less than or within 6 months of their last treatment. Fifty-four patients participated in this study, and 52 were assessable for response. Tumor histology included leiomyosarcoma (26 nonuterine, 15 uterine), liposarcoma (n = 11), GIST (n = 7), synovial sarcoma (n = 6), malignant fibrous histiocytoma (n = 6), fibrosarcoma (n = 7), and other (n = 22). Patients received a median of three cycles of ET-743. Results revealed two partial responses, four minor responses, and nine who had stable disease. Median progression-free survival was 1.9 months (range, 0.69–17.9 months), and 24% of patients were progression-free at 6 months. At 2 years, 30% of patients were alive, with an overall median survival of 12.8 months. Two patients died of treatment-related causes, renal failure, and febrile neutropenia, and rhabdomyolysis and decompensated cirrhosis, respectively. Both deaths were attributed to protocol eligibility violations. Fifty percent of patients had reversible grade 3 to 4 elevations in aspartate aminotransferase or alanine aminotransferase, and 61% of patients had grade 3 to 4 neutropenia, with six episodes of febrile neutropenia. Four percent (95% CI, 0.5%–12.8%) of patients had a partial response rate, and an additional 25% of patients had either a minor response or stable disease. Furthermore, three patients who received ET-743 were subsequently rendered tumor-free after undergoing surgery. This study shows that a 24-hour continuous infusion of ET-743 is a feasible option for patients with pretreated, progressing soft-tissue sarcomas [27]. ET-743 warrants additional development as a single agent or in combination in this subset of patients.

A second multicenter phase 2 and pharmacokinetic study of ET-743 was performed in patients who had progressive soft-tissue sarcomas refractory to chemotherapy, which more or less confirmed the results of the first trial [28]. As in the first trial, patients received ET-743 as a 24-hour continuous intravenous at a dose of 1500 $\mu g/m^2$ every 3 weeks, and pharmacokinetic studies were performed. This was a slightly smaller study with only 36 participants. Tumor histology included leiomyosarcoma (n = 13), liposarcoma (n = 10), synovial sarcoma (n = 6), malignant schwannoma (n = 2), and other (n = 5). The overall response rate was 8% (95% CI, 2% –23%), with one complete response and two partial responses. Responses lasted up 20 months. In addition, two patients had minor responses, for an overall clinical benefit of 14%. As in the previous study, the most common significant toxicities included grade 3 to 4 neutropenia (34% of patients) and grade 3 to 4 transaminitis (26% of patients). One-year estimates for time to progression and overall survival rates are 9% (95% CI, 3%–27%) and 53% (95% CI, 39%–73%), respectively. The pharmacokinetics were consistent with previous phase 1 study findings. The histologies with the most promising response to ET-743 included leiomyosarcoma and liposarcoma [28].

With the results of the above study as a guide, another multicenter phase 2 study of ET-743 was undertaken, but this time two different dosing schedules were evaluated in just two different histologies: leiomyosarcoma and liposarcoma [29]. To be eligible for this study, patients had to be refractory to conventional doxorubicin and ifosfamide chemotherapy. The two different dosing schedules of ET-743 included either administration as a 3-hour IV infusion given weekly for three consecutive weeks with the fourth week off on a 28-day cycle (arm A) or administration as a 24-hour IV infusion once every 3 weeks (arm B). At the time the initial results of this trial were reported, 60 patients had been accrued and 29 patients were eligible for evaluation. Out of the 15 patients on arm A, eight had progressed or died, three had stable disease at two cycles, and four had either a partial response or stable disease at four cycles. Similar results were seen on arm B; out of 14 patients, five had progressed or died, five had stable disease at two cycles, and four had a partial response or stable disease at four cycles. This study demonstrates that ET-743 at either dosing schedule is an active agent in this subgroup of patients with refractory leiomyosarcoma or liposarcoma [29].

Bortezomib

One of the new targets for novel drug therapy is the proteosome, an enzyme present in all human cells, which has a central role in the proteolytic degradation of most intracellular proteins. Some of the key proteins modulated by the proteosome are those involved in cell cycle regulation and gene expression [30]. For this reason, proteosome inhibitors, such as bortezomib (PS-341), have been shown to be active in cancer. A phase 2 multicenter trial is currently evaluating bortezomib in a two-arm study in adult patients who have metastatic or recurrent sarcomas, with either Ewing's sarcoma, osteogenic sarcoma, or rhabdomyosarcoma, or other STSs. The primary endpoint of this study is the determination of response rate. Bortezomib is given in this trial at a dosage of 1.5 mg/m^2 intravenous push twice weekly, 2 weeks on, 1 week off. At the time the preliminary results of this trial were reported, no patients had been enrolled on arm A, and 13 patients were enrolled on arm B with histologies including: five patients who had liposarcoma, two who had leiomyosarcoma, two who had alveolar soft parts sarcoma, and two who had malignant fibrous histiocytoma. Adverse effects have included constipation/abdominal pain, myalgias, persistent neuropathy, and fatigue. Of 11 evaluable patients, the best response is progression in seven patients, stable disease in two, and too early for evaluation in two others. At the time these preliminary results were presented, accrual was ongoing [31]. An update of this trial will most likely give a better idea if bortezomib will have a role in the treatment of STSs.

9-Nitrocamptothecin

We performed a two-arm phase 2 trial of 9-nitrocamptothecin (9-NC), an oral topoisomerase I inhibitor, to define the response rates in patients who have gastrointestinal (GI) leiomyosarcomas and other STSs. 9-NC was administered orally at 1.5 $mg/m^2/d$ for 5 days every week. A group of 56 patients (30 women and 26 men) that had a median age of 55 years was enrolled in this study. Seventeen patients were enrolled on the GI leiomyosarcoma arm; however, only one minor response lasting less than 8 weeks was noted, and so this arm was terminated. Thirty-nine patients were entered on the other STS arm. Of these patients, three achieved a partial response (response rate, 8%) for durations of 4, 6, and 13 months, respectively. Fourteen patients had stable disease for a median of 4 months (range, 2–8 months). Two patients died of disease during the first 2 months. Four other patients required hospitalization for nausea, vomiting, and dehydration. Other toxicities included diarrhea, fatigue, anorexia, neutropenia, and thrombocytopenia. 9-NC was found to be well tolerated but inactive in GI leiomyosarcoma, and to have minimal activity in previously treated patients who had STS [32].

Pegylated liposomal doxorubicin

Historically, adriamycin has been part of the cornerstone of treatment for advanced STSs. In an attempt to improve the antitumor activity of adriamycin and reduce its dose-limiting toxicities, new formulations have been developed. One such formulation is pegylated liposomal doxorubicin, a liposomal formulation of doxorubicin, that is sterically stabilized by coupling segments of polyethylene glycol onto the liposomal surface. The hope is that higher doses can be delivered safely and more efficiently [33].

A randomized phase 2 trial by the EORTC Soft Tissue and Bone Sarcoma Group compared pegylated liposomal doxorubicin (Caelyx; Schering-Plough, Kenilworth, New Jersey) with doxorubicin in the treatment of advanced or metastatic STS [34]. In this prospective trial, 94 eligible patients who had advanced STS were treated, 50 with Caelyx 50 mg/m^2 by a 1-hour IV infusion every 4 weeks and 44 with doxorubicin, 75 mg/m^2 by an IV bolus every 3 weeks. Histologic subtypes were evenly matched. Caelyx was significantly less myelosuppressive; only three (6%) patients had grade 3 and 4 neutropenia compared with 33 (77%) patients on doxorubicin. Febrile neutropenia occurred in seven (16%) patients given doxorubicin, but only one (2%) patient given Caelyx. Alopecia was much more common in patients given doxorubicin compared with Caelyx, 37 (86%) and 3 (6%) patients, respectively. The major toxicity with Caelyx was to the skin in the form of palmar-plantar erythrodysesthesia. The response rates for Caelyx were as follows: one complete response and four partial responses, for an overall response rate of 10%. Response rates were similar for Adriamycin: one complete and three partial responses, with an overall response rate of 9%. The reason for the low response rate in this study is unclear, but it may be partly because of the large number of gastrointestinal stromal tumors. The investigators propose further investigation of Caelyx in combination with other agents such as ifosfamide [34].

The combination of pegylated liposomal doxorubicin and paclitaxel in patients who have advanced STS has recently been investigated in a phase 2 study by the Hellenic Cooperative Oncology Group [33]. This multicenter study evaluated the safety and efficacy of pegylated liposomal doxorubicin and paclitaxel as first-line treatment in patients who have advanced STSs. A total of 42 patients who have either locally advanced or metastatic STSs and a median age of 54 years were treated with pegylated liposomal doxorubicin 45 mg/m^2 and paclitaxel 150 mg/m^2 every 28 days for a total of six cycles. The most common histologic subtypes were leiomyosarcomas (43%), malignant fibrous histiocytomas (14%), and liposarcomas (12%). Responses consisted of one (2%) complete response, six (14%) partial responses, and 14 (33%) patients who had stable disease. At a median follow-up of 41.5 months, median time to progression was 5.7 months and median overall survival was 13.2 months. Grade 3 to 4 toxicities included neutropenia (17%), anemia (15%), neurotoxicity (5%), and palmar-plantar erythrodysesthesia (9%). This combination of pegylated liposomal doxorubicin and paclitaxel appears safe and generally well tolerated with modest efficacy as first-line treatment in patients who have advanced soft-tissue sarcomas [33].

Oblimersen

For those patients who have GIST who never responded to imatinib and for those patients who stopped responding to imatinib after an initial response, new treatment strategies are desperately needed. Another agent that is being looked at for such patients is oblimersen (Genasense; Genta, Berkeley Heights, New Jersey), an 18-mer phosphorothioate oligonucleotide that targets the first six codons of the bcl-2 mRNA open reading frame to form a DNA/RNA duplex. RNase H recognizes the duplex, cleaves the bcl-2 mRNA strand, and renders the message nontranslatable. Bcl-2 mRNA fragments are subsequently destroyed by ribonucleases. Preclinical studies have established that bcl-2 mRNA and protein are specifically down-regulated by oblimersen [35–37]. Multiple phase 1 and 2 clinical studies in patients who have advanced cancer have established the safety of oblimersen, used either alone or in combination with other cytotoxic chemotherapy (including imatinib) [38–40].

A multicenter phase 2A study to determine the safety and efficacy of oblimersen combined with imatinib mesylate in patients who have refractory or relapsed GISTs is under development and should be open to accrual in the near future. Bcl-2 overexpression has been observed in GISTs and may mediate resistance to imatinib by inhibiting apoptosis. Patients will continue to take imatinib while on this trial as there is concern that withdrawal of this drug may lead to acceleration of tumor growth [41]. Oblimersen will be administered at a dose of 7 mg/kg/d by continuous IV infusion using an ambulatory infusion pump for 14 consecutive days on a 28-day cycle.

References

[1] Patel SR, Gandhi V, Jenkins J, et al. Phase II clinical investigation of gemcitabine in advanced soft tissue sarcomas and window evaluation of dose rate on gemcitabine triphosphate accumulation. J Clin Oncol 2001;19:3483–9.

[2] Hensley ML, Maki R, Venkatraman E, et al. Gemcitabine and docetaxel in patients with unresectable leiomyosarcoma: results of a phase II trial. J Clin Oncol 2002;20:2824–31.

[3] Hensley ML, Anderson S, Soslow R, et al. Activity of gemcitabine plus docetaxel in leiomyosarcoma (LMS) and other histologies: report of an expanded phase II trial [abstract 9010]. 2004 ASCO Annual Meeting Proceedings 2004;22:820s.

[4] Look K, Sandler A, Blessing J, et al. Phase II trial of gemcitabine as second-line chemotherapy of uterine leiomyosarcoma: a Gynecologic Oncology Group (GOG) study. Gynecol Oncol 2004;92:644–7.

[5] Morgan J, George S, Desai J, et al. Phase II study of gemcitabine/vinorelbine (GV) as first or second line chemotherapy in patients with metastatic soft tissue sarcoma (STS) [abstract 9009]. 2004 ASCO Annual Meeting Proceedings 2004;22:820s.

[6] Druker B, Talpez M, Resta D. Efficacy and safety of a specific inhibitor of the BCR-ABL tyrosine kinase in chronic myeloid leukemia. N Engl J Med 2001;344:1031–7.

[7] Joensuu H, Roberts P, Sarlomo-Rikala M, et al. Effect of the tyrosine kinase inhibitor STI571 in a patient with a metastatic gastrointestinal stromal tumor. N Engl J Med 2001; 344:1052–6.

[8] van Oosterom AT, Judson I, Verweij J, et al. Safety and efficacy of imatinib (STI571) in metastatic gastrointestinal stromal tumours: a phase I study. Lancet 2001;358:1421–3.

[9] Demetri GD, von Mehren M, Blanke CD, et al. Efficacy and safety of imatinib mesylate in advanced gastrointestinal stromal tumors. N Engl J Med 2002;347:472–80.

[10] von Mehren M, Blanke C, Joensuu H, et al. High Incidence of durable responses induced by imatinib mesylate (Gleevec) in patients with unresectable and metastatic gastrointestinal stromal tumors (GISTs) [abstract 1608]. Proceedings of the American Society of Clinical Oncology. Orlando (FL): American Society of Clinical Oncology; 2002. p. 403a.

[11] Verweij J, van Oosterom A, Blay J, et al. Imatinib mesylate (STI-571 Glivec, Gleevec) is an active agent for gastrointestinal stromal tumours, but does not yield responses in other soft-tissue sarcomas that are unselected for a molecular target: results from an EORTC Soft Tissue and Bone Sarcoma Group phase II study. Eur J Cancer 2003;39:2006–11.

[12] Benjamin RS, Rankin C, Fletcher C, et al. Phase III dose-randomized study of imatinib mesylate (STI-571) for GIST: Intergroup S0033 early results [abstract 3271]. Chicago: American Society of Clinical Oncology; 2003. p. 814.

[13] Rankin C, von Mehren M, Blanke C, et al. Dose effect of imatinib (IM) in patients (pts) with metastatic GIST—Phase III Sarcoma Group Study S0033 [abstract 9005]. Annual Meeting Proceedings of the American Society of Clinical Oncology 2004;23:815.

[14] Verweij J, Casali PG, Zalcberg J, et al. Progression-free survival in gastrointestinal stromal tumours with high-dose imatinib: randomised trial. Lancet 2004;364:1127–34.

[14a] Debiec-Rychter M, Cools J, Dumez H, et al. Mechanisms of resistance to imatinib mesylate in gastrointestinal stromal tumors and activity of the PKC 412 inhibitor against imatinib-resistant mutants. Gastroenterology 2005;128:270–9.

[15] Demetri G, Desai J, Fletcher JA, et al. SU11248, a multi-targeted tyrosine kinase inhibitor, can overcome imatinib (IM) resistance caused by diverse genomic mechanisms in patients (pts) with metastatic gastrointestinal stromal tumor (GIST) [abstract 3001]. 2004 ASCO Annual Meeting Proceedings 2004;23:195.

[16] van Oosterom A, Dumez H, Desai J, et al. Combination signal transduction inhibition: a phase I/II trial of the oral mTOR-inhibitor everolimus (E,RAD001) and imatinib mesylate (IM) in patients (pts) with gastrointestinal stromal tumor (GIST) refractory to IM [abstract 3002]. 2004 ASCO Annual Meeting Proceedings 2004;23:195.

[17] Shimizu A, O'Brien KP, Sjoblom T, et al. The dermatofibrosarcoma protuberans-associated

collagen type Ialpha1/platelet-derived growth factor (PDGF) B-chain fusion gene generates a transforming protein that is processed to functional PDGF-BB. Cancer Res 1999;59: 3719–23.
[18] Rubin BP, Schuetze SM, Eary JF, et al. Molecular targeting of platelet-derived growth factor B by imatinib mesylate in a patient with metastatic dermatofibrosarcoma protuberans. J Clin Oncol 2002;20:3586–91.
[19] Maki RG, Awan RA, Dixon RH, et al. Differential sensitivity to imatinib of 2 patients with metastatic sarcoma arising from dermatofibrosarcoma protuberans. Int J Cancer 2002;100: 623–6.
[20] McArthur G, Demetri G, Heinrich MC, et al. Molecular and clinical analysis of response to imatinib for locally advanced dermatofibrosarcoma protuberans. Eur J Cancer 2004;8(Suppl 2):12 [abstract 28].
[21] Mace J, Sybil Biermann J, Sondak V, et al. Response of extraabdominal desmoid tumors to therapy with imatinib mesylate. Cancer 2002;95:2373–9.
[22] Baker L, Wathen K, Chugh R, et al. Activity of imatinib mesylate in desmoid tumors: interim analysis of a Sarcoma Alliance for Research thru Collaboration (SARC) phase II trial [abstract 9013]. 2004 ASCO Annual Meeting Proceedings 2004;22:821s.
[23] Chugh R, Thomas D, Wathen K, et al. Imatinib mesylate in soft tissue and bone sarcomas: interim results of a Sarcoma Alliance for Research thru Collaboration (SARC) phase II trial [abstract 9001]. 2004 ASCO Annual Meeting Proceedings 2004;22:818s.
[24] Casper ES, Waltzman RJ, Schwartz GK, et al. Phase II trial of paclitaxel in patients with soft-tissue sarcoma. Cancer Invest 1998;16:442–6.
[25] Fata F, O'Reilly E, Ilson D, et al. Paclitaxel in the treatment of patients with angiosarcoma of the scalp or face. Cancer 1999;86:2034–7.
[26] Delaloge S, Yovine A, Taamma A, et al. Ecteinascidin-743: a marine-derived compound in advanced, pretreated sarcoma patients–preliminary evidence of activity. J Clin Oncol 2001; 19:1248–55.
[27] Yovine A, Riofrio M, Blay JY, et al. Phase II study of ecteinascidin-743 in advanced pretreated soft tissue sarcoma patients. J Clin Oncol 2004;22:890–9.
[28] Garcia-Carbonero R, Supko JG, Manola J, et al. Phase II and pharmacokinetic study of ecteinascidin 743 in patients with progressive sarcomas of soft tissues refractory to chemotherapy. J Clin Oncol 2004;22:1480–90.
[29] Samuels B, Rushing D, Chawla S, et al. Randomized phase II study of trabectedin (ET-743) given by two different dosing schedules in patients (pts) with leiomyosarcoma (LMS) or liposarcoma (LPS) refractory to conventional doxorubicin and ifosfamide chemotherapy [abstract 9000]. 2004 ASCO Annual Meeting Proceedings 2004;22:818s.
[30] Elliott PJ, Ross JS. The proteasome: a new target for novel drug therapies. Am J Clin Pathol 2001;116:637–46.
[31] Maki R, Kraft A, Demetri G, et al. A phase II multicenter study of proteasome inhibitor PS-341 (LDP-341, bortezomib) for untreated recurrent or metastatic soft tissue sarcoma (STS); CTEP study 1757 [abstract 3291]. 2003 ASCO Annual Meeting Proceedings 2003;22:819.
[32] Patel SR, Beach J, Papadopoulos N, et al. Results of a 2-arm Phase II study of 9-nitrocamptothecin in patients with advanced soft-tissue sarcomas. Cancer 2003;97:2848–52.
[33] Bafaloukos D, Papadimitriou C, Linardou H, et al. Combination of pegylated liposomal doxorubicin (PLD) and paclitaxel in patients with advanced soft tissue sarcoma: a phase II study of the Hellenic Cooperative Oncology Group. Br J Cancer 2004;91:1639–44.
[34] Judson I, Radford JA, Harris M, et al. Randomised phase II trial of pegylated liposomal doxorubicin (DOXIL/CAELYX) versus doxorubicin in the treatment of advanced or metastatic soft tissue sarcoma: a study by the EORTC Soft Tissue and Bone Sarcoma Group. Eur J Cancer 2001;37:870–7.
[35] Kitada S, Miyashita T, Tanaka S, et al. Investigations of antisense oligonucleotides targeted against bcl-2 RNAs. Antisense Res Dev 1993;3:157–69.
[36] Cotter FE, Johnson P, Hall P, et al. Antisense oligonucleotides suppress B-cell lymphoma growth in a SCID-hu mouse model. Oncogene 1994;9:3049–55.

[37] Jansen B, Schlagbauer-Wadl H, Brown BD, et al. bcl-2 antisense therapy chemosensitizes human melanoma in SCID mice. Nat Med 1998;4:232–4.

[38] Morris MJ, Tong WP, Cordon-Cardo C, et al. Phase I trial of BCL-2 antisense oligonucleotide (G3139) administered by continuous intravenous infusion in patients with advanced cancer. Clin Cancer Res 2002;8:679–83.

[39] Tolcher AW, Kuhn J, Schwartz G, et al. A phase I pharmacokinetic and biological correlative study of oblimersen sodium (genasense, g3139), an antisense oligonucleotide to the bcl-2 mRNA, and of docetaxel in patients with hormone-refractory prostate cancer. Clin Cancer Res 2004;10:5048–57.

[40] Rudin CM, Kozloff M, Hoffman PC, et al. Phase I study of G3139, a bcl-2 antisense oligonucleotide, combined with carboplatin and etoposide in patients with small-cell lung cancer. J Clin Oncol 2004;22:1110–7.

[41] Demetri G, Benjamin R, Blanke CD, et al. NCCN task force report: optimal management of patients with gastrointestinal stromal tumor (GIST)—expansion and update of NCCN clinical practice guidelines. Journal of the National Comprehensive Cancer Network 2004;2(Suppl 1): S1–26.

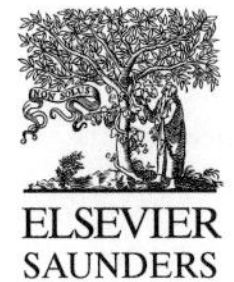

ELSEVIER
SAUNDERS

Hematol Oncol Clin N Am
19 (2005) 591–596

HEMATOLOGY/
ONCOLOGY
CLINICS OF
NORTH AMERICA

Index

Note: Page numbers of article titles are in **boldface** type.

doi:10.1016/S0889-8588(05)00057-2

K

L

M

N

O

P

R

S

Changing Your Address?

Make sure your subscription changes too! When you notify us of your new address, you can help make our job easier by including an exact copy of your Clinics label number with your old address (see illustration below.) This number identifies you to our computer system and will speed the processing of your address change. Please be sure this label number accompanies your old address and your corrected address—you can send an old Clinics label with your number on it or just copy it exactly and send it to the address listed below.

We appreciate your help in our attempt to give you continuous coverage. Thank you.

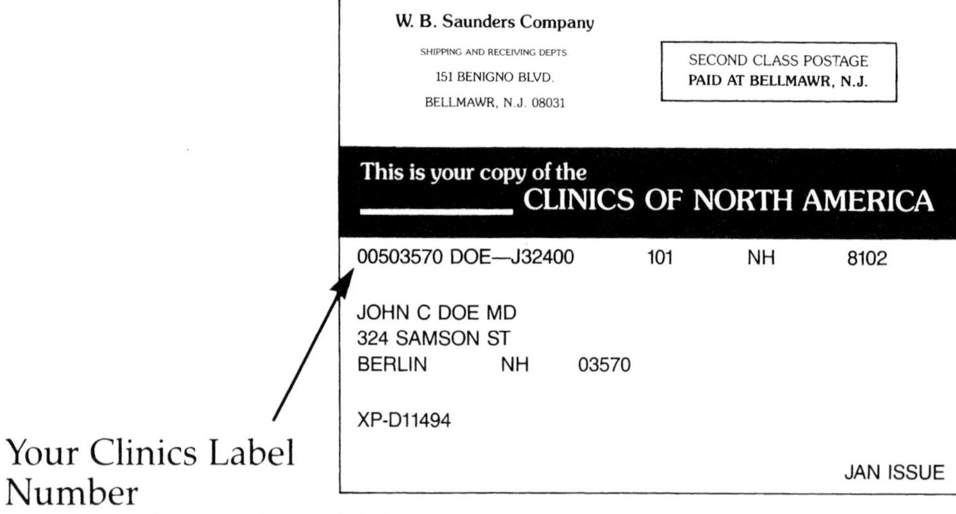

Your Clinics Label Number

Copy it exactly or send your label
along with your address to:
W.B. Saunders Company, Customer Service
Orlando, FL 32887-4800
Call Toll Free 1-800-654-2452

Please allow four to six weeks for delivery of new subscriptions and for processing address changes.